Sulfur-Containing Marine Bioactives

Sulfur-Containing Marine Bioactives

Editor

Anna Palumbo

MDPI • Basel • Beijing • Wuhan • Barcelona • Belgrade • Manchester • Tokyo • Cluj • Tianjin

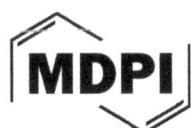

Editor
Anna Palumbo
Stazione Zoologica Anton Dohrn,
Department of Biology and
Evolution of Marine Organisms
Italy

Editorial Office
MDPI
St. Alban-Anlage 66
4052 Basel, Switzerland

This is a reprint of articles from the Special Issue published online in the open access journal *Marine Drugs* (ISSN 1660-3397) (available at: https://www.mdpi.com/journal/marinedrugs/special_issues/Sulfur-Containing_Marine_Bioactives).

For citation purposes, cite each article independently as indicated on the article page online and as indicated below:

LastName, A.A.; LastName, B.B.; LastName, C.C. Article Title. *Journal Name* **Year**, *Volume Number*, Page Range.

ISBN 978-3-0365-0490-2 (Hbk)
ISBN 978-3-0365-0491-9 (PDF)

© 2021 by the authors. Articles in this book are Open Access and distributed under the Creative Commons Attribution (CC BY) license, which allows users to download, copy and build upon published articles, as long as the author and publisher are properly credited, which ensures maximum dissemination and a wider impact of our publications.

The book as a whole is distributed by MDPI under the terms and conditions of the Creative Commons license CC BY-NC-ND.

Contents

About the Editor . . . . **vii**

Preface to "Sulfur-Containing Marine Bioactives" . . . . **ix**

Geovanna Parra-Riofrío, Jorge García-Márquez, Virginia Casas-Arrojo, Eduardo Uribe-Tapia and Roberto Teófilo Abdala-Díaz
Antioxidant and Cytotoxic Effects on Tumor Cells of Exopolysaccharides from *Tetraselmis suecica* (Kylin) Butcher Grown Under Autotrophic and Heterotrophic Conditions
Reprinted from: *Mar. Drugs* **2020**, *18*, 534, doi:10.3390/md18110534 . . . . **1**

Cátia Vilas-Boas, Francisca Carvalhal, Beatriz Pereira, Sílvia Carvalho, Emília Sousa, Madalena M. M. Pinto, Maria José Calhorda, Vitor Vasconcelos, Joana R. Almeida, Elisabete R. Silva and Marta Correia-da-Silva
One Step Forward towards the Development of Eco-Friendly Antifouling Coatings: Immobilization of a Sulfated Marine-Inspired Compound
Reprinted from: *Mar. Drugs* **2020**, *18*, 489, doi:10.3390/md18100489 . . . . **25**

Alfonsina Milito, Ida Orefice, Arianna Smerilli, Immacolata Castellano, Alessandra Napolitano, Christophe Brunet and Anna Palumbo
Insights into the Light Response of *Skeletonema marinoi*: Involvement of Ovothiol
Reprinted from: *Mar. Drugs* **2020**, *18*, 477, doi:10.3390/md18090477 . . . . **43**

Emiliano Manzo, Laura Fioretto, Carmela Gallo, Marcello Ziaco, Genoveffa Nuzzo, Giuliana D'Ippolito, Assunta Borzacchiello, Antonio Fabozzi, Raffaele De Palma and Angelo Fontana
Preparation, Supramolecular Aggregation and Immunological Activity of the Bona Fide Vaccine Adjuvant Sulfavant S
Reprinted from: *Mar. Drugs* **2020**, *18*, 451, doi:10.3390/md18090451 . . . . **61**

Pilar Garcia-Jimenez, Sara R. Mantesa and Rafael R. Robaina
Expression of Genes Related to Carrageenan Synthesis during Carposporogenesis of the Red Seaweed *Grateloupia imbricata*
Reprinted from: *Mar. Drugs* **2020**, *18*, 432, doi:10.3390/md18090432 . . . . **73**

Shadi Khodamoradi, Marc Stadler, Joachim Wink and Frank Surup
Litoralimycins A and B, New Cytotoxic Thiopeptides from *Streptomonospora* sp. M2
Reprinted from: *Mar. Drugs* **2020**, *18*, 280, doi:10.3390/md18060280 . . . . **87**

Philipp Dörschmann, Georg Kopplin, Johann Roider and Alexa Klettner
Effects of Sulfated Fucans from *Laminaria hyperborea* Regarding VEGF Secretion, Cell Viability, and Oxidative Stress and Correlation with Molecular Weight
Reprinted from: *Mar. Drugs* **2019**, *17*, 548, doi:10.3390/md17100548 . . . . **97**

He Ma, Peiju Qiu, Huixin Xu, Ximing Xu, Meng Xin, Yanyan Chu, Huashi Guan, Chunxia Li and Jinbo Yang
The Inhibitory Effect of Propylene Glycol Alginate Sodium Sulfate on Fibroblast Growth Factor 2-Mediated Angiogenesis and Invasion in Murine Melanoma B16-F10 Cells In Vitro
Reprinted from: *Mar. Drugs* **2019**, *17*, 257, doi:10.3390/md17050257 . . . . **111**

About the Editor

Anna Palumbo obtained her degree in Biology in 1976. In 1980 she became Research Scientist, in 1992 Senior Scientist, and in 2007 Research Director at the Stazione Zoologica Anton Dohrn. She has spent some periods abroad at INSERM and INSA in France and as a visiting scientist at NIH, Bethesda and at MRC, Edinburgh. Her research interests are mainly focused on marine organisms. In particular, she investigated the biosynthesis, signaling, and roles of nitric oxide in relation to the cuttlefish defense system and ascidian development. More recently, her research interests have been focused on understanding how marine organisms are responding and might adapt to the increasing pressure exerted by climatic changes and human activities. The actions of some environmental conditions (acidification, toxic bloom, and contaminants such as microplastics) on marine organisms at different life phases have been examined by laboratory or field experiments. Moreover, great attention has also been focused on the biological properties of marine bioactive molecules, with the aim of developing pharmacological applications.

Preface to "Sulfur-Containing Marine Bioactives"

This Special Issue, entitled "Sulfur-Containing Marine Bioactives", highlights the most recent findings related to the biological function of some marine sulfur metabolites and their effect on different cellular systems, with a focus on potential pharmacological properties.

Milito et al. show the involvement of ovothiols, which are histidine-derived thiols, in the light-dependent response of the diatom *Skeletonema marinoi*. Ovothiol biosynthesis is induced by high sinusoidal light mimicking natural conditions. Garcia-Jimenez et al. provide insights into the involvement of the sulfation and desulfation of galactan backbone in carrageenan synthesis in the red seaweed *Grateloupia imbricata* during thalli development and cystocarp maturation.

Parra-Riofrio et al. report that the microalga *Tetraselmis suecica* produces exopolysaccharides containing sulfate at higher yields when grown under heterotrophic conditions. These exopolysaccharides show antioxidant and cytotoxic effects on tumor cells, suggesting their possible use as nutraceuticals. Dorschmann et al. purify three sulfated fucans at different molecular weights from the brown alga *Laminaria hyperborea* and investigate their effects on cell viability, oxidative stress protection, and vascular endothelial growth factor secretion in ocular cells. The potential use of these compounds in the treatment of ocular diseases, such as age-related macular degeneration, is envisaged. Ma et al. investigate the effect of propylene glycol alginate sodium sulfate, obtained from the alginate polysaccharide of *Laminaria*, on FGF2-mediated angiogenesis and invasion in melanoma cells. Their results suggest its involvement in the regulation of the tumor microenvironment. Khodamoradi et al. characterize two new thiopeptides, litoralimycins A and B, from a new actinomycetes bacterium, with one exhibiting strong cytotoxic activity.

Inspired by some marine sulfur compounds, Manzo et al. report that the immunological potency of a novel class of vaccine adjuvants, namely Sulfavants, is dependent on the supramolecular aggregation states. Vilas-Boas et al. synthesize coatings containing immobilized gallic acid persulfate that exhibit an anti-settlement effect against *Mytilus galloprovincialis* larvae.

Anna Palumbo
Editor

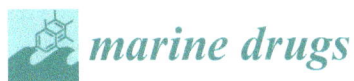

Article

Antioxidant and Cytotoxic Effects on Tumor Cells of Exopolysaccharides from *Tetraselmis suecica* (Kylin) Butcher Grown Under Autotrophic and Heterotrophic Conditions

Geovanna Parra-Riofrío [1,2,*], Jorge García-Márquez [3], Virginia Casas-Arrojo [4], Eduardo Uribe-Tapia [2] and Roberto Teófilo Abdala-Díaz [4,*]

1. Doctorado en Acuicultura, Programa Cooperativo Universidad de Chile, Universidad Católica del Norte, Pontificia Universidad Católica de Valparaíso, Valparaíso 2340000, Chile
2. Departamento de Acuicultura, Facultad de Ciencias del Mar, Universidad Católica del Norte, Larrondo 1281, Coquimbo, Chile; euribe@ucn.cl
3. Department of Microbiology, Faculty of Sciences, University of Malaga, 29071 Malaga, Spain; j.garcia@uma.es
4. Instituto de Biotecnología y Desarrollo Azul (IBYDA), Departamento de Ecología y Geología, Facultad de Ciencias, Universidad de Málaga, 29071 Málaga, Spain; virginiac@uma.es
* Correspondence: gbparrar@gmail.com (G.P.-R.); abdala@uma.es (R.T.A.-D.); Tel.: +56-966960044 (G.P.-R.); +34-952136652 (R.T.A.-D.)

Received: 27 September 2020; Accepted: 25 October 2020; Published: 26 October 2020

Abstract: Marine microalgae produce extracellular metabolites such as exopolysaccharides (EPS) with potentially beneficial biological applications to human health, especially antioxidant and antitumor properties, which can be increased with changes in crop trophic conditions. This study aimed to develop the autotrophic and heterotrophic culture of *Tetraselmis suecica* (Kylin) Butcher in order to increase EPS production and to characterize its antioxidant activity and cytotoxic effects on tumor cells. The adaptation of autotrophic to heterotrophic culture was carried out by progressively reducing the photoperiod and adding glucose. EPS extraction and purification were performed. EPS were characterized by Fourier-transform infrared spectroscopy and gas chromatography-mass spectrometry. The antioxidant capacity of EPS was analyzed by the 2,2'-azino-bis (3-ethylbenzothiazoline-6-sulphonic acid) (ABTS) method, and the antitumor capacity was measured by the 3-(4,5-dimethylthiazol-2-yl)-2,5-diphenyltetrazolium bromide (MTT) assay, showing high activity on human leukemia, breast and lung cancer cell lines. Although total EPS showed no cytotoxicity, acidic EPS showed cytotoxicity over the gingival fibroblasts cell line. Heterotrophic culture has advantages over autotrophic, such as increasing EPS yield, higher antioxidant capacity of the EPS and, to the best of our knowledge, this is the first probe that *T. suecica* EPS have cytotoxic effects on tumor cells; therefore, they could offer greater advantages as possible natural nutraceuticals for the pharmaceutical industry.

Keywords: *Tetraselmis suecica*; autotrophic culture; heterotrophic culture; exopolysaccharides; antioxidant capacity; cytotoxic effects on tumor cells

1. Introduction

Microalgae can develop in autotrophic, mixotrophic and heterotrophic conditions due to their physiological characteristics and plasticity of adaptation on our planet [1], differentiating them by the type of energy and the source of carbon to be used [2]. The cultivation of microalgae is mostly performed in autotrophy using light as an energy source, which is transformed by photosynthesis into chemical energy for the storage of polysaccharides and lipids [3,4].

In a heterotrophic culture, microalgae have the ability to grow and metabolize organic carbon sources with limited irradiance [5], changing their metabolism to generate energy by breathing or using an organic substrate under heterotrophic conditions [6]. It has several advantages over an autotrophic crop: (i) it does not require lighting, (ii) high biomass yield, (iii) high growth rates and (iv) increased synthesis of metabolites of scientific and biotechnological interest [5–7]. These metabolites depend on changes in culture media; therefore, optimization of organic carbon, macronutrient and micronutrient concentrations is sought in order to obtain the best yields in terms of productivity and biomass [1,8].

Crop types and systems provide advances both for the production of biomass with high nutritional value and economic viability and for the search, extraction and characterization of new products [9,10]. Heterotrophic culture has a potential market for the production of high-value metabolites with respect to autotrophic crops: (i) lipids with four times higher content of polyunsaturated fatty acids (PUFAs) than those cultured in autotrophic conditions [11–13], (ii) accumulation of up to 45% by dry weight of carbohydrates [11,14,15], (iii) a higher percentage of proteins for the biomass [16] and (iv) pigments (lutein and phycocyanin) with balanced C/N ratios and astaxanthin with limiting nitrogen [17–19].

Tetraselmis suecica is a marine green microalga widely used in aquaculture as live food for rotifers and copepods or Artemia in hatcheries [20]. This microalga can be cultivated in autotrophic and heterotrophic conditions [21]. It has antibacterial activity [22,23], probiotic properties [24] and has been proposed as a source of vitamin E for humans [25]. *T. suecica* produces exopolysaccharides [26]; however, their structural characteristics and biotechnological applications in human health remain unknown.

Polysaccharides are high-molecular weight molecules that contain repetitive structural units—monosaccharides- joined by glucosidic bonds, forming linear or branched structures. This structural variability has biotechnological interest [27]. Its applications are promising due to its immunomodulatory, antimicrobial, antiviral, antioxidant and antitumoral capacities [28]. Algal polysaccharides are free radical scavengers and, therefore, have antioxidant effects and prevent oxidative damage in living organisms [29]. The antioxidant activity of polysaccharides has been related to the presence of sulfates and uronic acids in them [28,30]. In this sense, in vitro antiproliferative activity in human cancer cells lines [31] and in vivo inhibition of Graffi myeloid tumor growth in hamsters [32] have been demonstrated with marine algal polysaccharides. Therefore, the prospecting of natural-origin compounds such as polysaccharides is a source for the prevention of diseases that counteract the toxic effects of synthetic compounds.

The aim of this work was to develop the crop of *T. suecica* under autotrophic and heterotrophic conditions, comparing the differences between the biochemical composition of the algal biomass and their yield exopolysaccharides (EPS). Furthermore, the functional groups, monosaccharides characterization and the antioxidant activity and cytotoxic effects on tumor cells and healthy cells of the exopolysaccharides were assessed.

2. Results and Discussion

2.1. Adaptation of Autotrophic to Heterotrophic Culture of T. suecica

The heterotrophic culture of *T. suecica* showed that cell density, cell concentration and biovolume were statistically higher in the heterotrophic culture ($p < 0.05$), while the cell volume was 17 times lower compared with the autotrophic culture ($p < 0.05$) (Table 1). The specific growth rate between autotrophic and heterotrophic cultures no showed statistic differences significantly (Table 1).

Table 1. Population parameter from autotrophic and heterotrophic cultures of *T. suecica* (mean ± SD; $n = 3$). Asterisks denote significant differences ($p < 0.05$, Student's *t*-test).

Population Parameter	Autotrophic	Heterotrophic
Cell density (cell mL^{-1})	$2.0 \times 10^6 \pm 1.6 \times 10^4$	$3.6 \times 10^7 \pm 7.7 \times 10^4$ *
Cell concentration (g L^{-1})	5.5 ± 0.5	10.2 ± 0.7 *
Specific growth rate (μ) (d^{-1})	0.3 ± 0.2	0.3 ± 0.2
Biovolume (μm^3 mL^{-1})	$8.8 \times 10^8 \pm 2.8 \times 10^8$	$1.2 \times 10^9 \pm 3.0 \times 10^8$ *
Cell volume (μm^3)	521 ± 33 *	30 ± 2

Azma et al. [12] obtained differences in the final cell concentration of *T. suecica* grown in autotrophy and heterotrophy. On the contrary, Day and Tsavalos [33] found no differences in the final cell concentration of *Tetraselmis* sp. between the two culture conditions. These variations could be due to growth in the absence of light, and the presence of organic substrates can change the metabolism and morphology of cells. In our investigation, glucose was used as the source of organic carbon, which generated high cellular concentrations due to the energy provided (2.8 kJ mol^{-1}), compared to the 0.8 kJ mol^{-1} for acetate used in Azma et al.'s [12] investigation.

The adaptation of autotrophic to heterotrophic culture was performed by the progressive reduction of the illumination times in the photoperiod, preserving the irradiance of the *T. suecica* cultures. However, Azma et al. [21] made a progressive decrease in lighting for *T. suecica* cultures with longer periods, adding a total of 1650 h compared to the present study, which was 1080 h for adaptation to heterotrophy, meaning 35% less hours of adaptation, which would be due to the different media used in cultivation. The Walne medium [34] used in Azma et al.'s [21] investigation contained concentrations of nitrate, phosphate, ethylenediaminetetraacetic acid (EDTA), zinc, molybdenum and manganese higher than F/2 used in the present study. Therefore, *T. suecica* has the ability to regulate its metabolism to achieve balanced growth in heterotrophic culture; this capability can be used to increase the production of metabolites of biotechnological interest.

2.2. Elemental Analysis of Autotrophic and Heterotrophic Biomass Cultures of T. suecica

Heterotrophic cultures of *T. suecica* showed higher carbon and nitrogen contents than those observed in autotrophy ($p < 0.05$; Table 2). The C/N ratio did not show statistical differences ($p > 0.05$) between both culture conditions (Table 2). The C/N ratio is a nutritional indicator of the microalgae. When N is low, the C/N ratio favors the biosynthesis and accumulation of carbohydrates [35]. However, Cheng et al. [36] mentioned that a C/N ratio higher than 10 allowed lipid accumulation in heterotrophic cultures. In our study, the high C/N ratio is favored for the accumulation of carbon, which will be used to increase the accumulation of lipids or carbohydrates.

Table 2. Total carbon (TC), total nitrogen (TN) content and C/N ratio in the biomass obtained from autotrophic and heterotrophic cultures of *T. suecica* (mean ± SD; $n = 3$). Asterisks denote significant differences ($p < 0.05$, Student's *t*-test).

Elemental Analysis (%)	Autotrophic	Heterotrophic
TC	25.7 ± 0.4	31.0 ± 0.1 *
TN	3.5 ± 0.2	4.3 ± 0.1 *
C/N	7.3 ± 0.2	7.2 ± 0.1

2.3. Biochemical Composition of Autotrophic and Heterotrophic Biomass Cultures of T. suecica

Heterotrophic cultures eliminate the light limitations that autotrophic cultures require, generating metabolic changes in microalgae, thus presenting variations in the biochemical composition of the biomass [6,7]. In our study, except for the percentage of ash ($p > 0.05$; Table 3), statistical differences in the biochemical composition of the autotrophic and heterotrophic cultures of *T. suecica* were found ($p < 0.05$; Table 3).

Table 3. Content of proteins, carbohydrates, lipids, ash and moisture in the biomass from autotrophic and heterotrophic cultures of *T. suecica* (% of dry weight (DW); mean ± SD; $n = 3$). Asterisks denote significant differences ($p < 0.05$, Student's *t*-test).

Biochemical Composition	Autotrophic	Heterotrophic
Proteins	16.76 ± 0.40	20.78 ± 0.14 *
Lipids	6.13 ± 0.12	7.96 ± 0.10 *
Carbohydrates	24.31 ± 0.32	28.18 ± 0.37 *
Ash	34.88 ± 0.08	33.07 ± 1.30
Moisture	17.93 ± 0.52 *	10.01 ± 1.16

The percentage of proteins in *T. suecica* statistically increased from 16.76% in autotrophy to 20.78% in heterotrophy ($p < 0.05$; Table 3). To the best of our knowledge, no studies regarding protein increase with respect to heterotrophic cultures has been reported; however, Cid et al. [37] showed that the addition of organic compounds to the culture medium increased the protein fraction in *T. suecica* mixotrophic cultures. El-Sheekh et al. [16] reported a significant increase in the percentage of proteins in mixotrophic cultures of *Chlorella vulgaris* and *Scenedesmus obliquus* with the addition of hydrolyzed wheat bran with respect to autotrophy. Canelli et al. [38] mentioned that heterotrophic cells convert the storage of cellular nitrogen into proteins, and when this nitrogen reserve is depleted, the consumption of intracellular carbon begins to increase the protein fraction. However, it is important to consider that a low C/N ratio induces protein accumulation [39].

In the case of lipids and carbohydrates, an increase in heterotrophic cultures of *T. suecica* is observed with respect to autotrophic cultures ($p < 0.05$; Table 3). In this sense, Azma et al. [12] observed that the heterotrophic culture of T. suecica presented a higher percentage of lipids with respect to the autotrophic culture. Furthermore, similar results were observed in heterotrophic cultures of *Chlorella protothecoides* and *C. vulgaris*, with lipid accumulations between 50–60% in the biomass [11,13]. Similar results of carbohydrate accumulation (>45%) in dry weight were observed for these microalgae species [15]. In our study, *T. suecica* increased in a greater percentage the carbohydrate content in relation to the lipids (Table 3). This could be because there was probably a depletion of N, observed by the high C/N index (Table 2). High growth rates in heterotrophic cultures led to nutrient depletion, decreasing cell division and allow them to accumulate carbon for the synthesis of lipids or carbohydrates [40]. Another factor could be the nitrogen deficiency, which induced the increase of lipids in the biomass [41]. Furthermore, Garcia-Ferris et al. [41] observed that, in periods of nitrogen starvation and heterotrophy, there was a decrease in the size of the chloroplast of *Euglena gracilis*. Additionally, in our study was observed a reduction in chloroplast size in the heterotrophic culture (data not shown). Similar results were observed by Gladue and Maxey [14] for *Tetraselmis* sp. in a heterotrophic culture.

2.4. Phenolic Compounds and Antioxidant Activity of Autotrophic and Heterotrophic Biomass Cultures of T. suecica

The phenol content of heterotrophic cultures of *T. suecica* was higher than autotrophic ($p < 0.05$; Table 4). To the best of our knowledge, our results are the first report of phenol content in heterotrophic cultures for the species under study. In heterotrophy, the mechanisms of accumulation and antioxidant response are related to nutritional stress [42]. Phenolic compounds are a defense mechanism against the excess of oxygen produced in photosynthesis, and the depletion of nutrients causes their accumulation [42]. Quiñones-Galvez et al. [43] showed that the heterotrophic cultivation of calluses of *Theobroma cacao* increased the phenolic content, due to the osmotic stress caused by the addition of glucose, favoring their synthesis and accumulation. This increase in phenolic compounds in heterotrophy was also observed for *C. vulgaris* and *S. obliquus* [44].

Table 4. Total phenolic content and antioxidant capacity measured by 2,2'-azino-bis (3-ethylbenzothiazoline-6-sulphonic acid) (ABTS) and 2,2-diphenyl-1-picrylhydrazyl (DPPH) assay in the biomass from autotrophic and heterotrophic cultures of *T. suecica* (mean ± SD; $n = 3$). Asterisks denote significant differences ($p < 0.05$, Student's *t*-test). TE: Trolox equivalents.

Culture	Phenols (mg Eq Phloroglucinol)	Antioxidant Activity	
		ABTS (μmol TE g^{-1} DW)	DPPH (μmol TE g^{-1} DW)
Autotrophic	3.88 ± 0.03	24.25 ± 0.70	3.49 ± 0.61
Heterotrophic	5.56 ± 0.10 *	80.17 ± 0.95 *	6.35 ± 0.91 *

The increase in antioxidant activity is due to the fact that the photosystem II of the cells produces reactive oxygen species (ROS), caused by the photosynthetic process [45]. However, in the adaptation of autotrophy to heterotrophy, photosystem II is reduced due to its low photosynthetic activity [46], decreasing the chlorophyll, carotene and phycobiliprotein contents, which are related to the nitrogen availability, and causing alterations in the electron transport system, leading to an increase in antioxidant activity [47,48].

The 2,2'-azino-bis (3-ethylbenzothiazoline-6-sulphonic acid) (ABTS) method measures hydrophilic and lipophilic antioxidants [49]. *T. suecica* increased the antioxidant activity measured by the ABTS method in heterotrophic cultures with respect to autotrophic ($p < 0.05$; Table 4). A positive correlation was found in the heterotrophic culture of *T. suecica* between ABTS and proteins, lipids, carbohydrates, total carbon (TC) and total nitrogen (TN) (Supplementary Table S1). This could be because the method also measures fat-soluble antioxidants (carotenoid, chlorophylls, vitamin E or tocopherols, PUFAs and polysaccharides) that are part of the biomass [49]. Although, in this study, no analysis of fatty acid composition was performed, an increase in the content of PUFAs in an heterotrophic cultivation of *T. suecica* has been reported [14,20], which would indicate that the increase in fatty acid composition is related to higher antioxidant activity [50].

The 2,2-diphenyl-1-picrylhydrazyl (DPPH) method measures the reducing capacity of the hydrophilic fraction of the compound [51]. In our study, *T. suecica* increased the antioxidant capacity in heterotrophic cultures with respect to autotrophic measured by the DPPH method ($p < 0.05$; Table 4). A positive correlation was found in the heterotrophic culture of *T. suecica* between the DPPH and phenolic content, lipids and TC (Supplementary Table S1). Therefore, it is attributed that the increase in antioxidant activity by the DPPH method is related to the content of phenols, because this assay performs a better measurement of hydrophilic compounds. Significant correlations have been observed in macroalgae [52]; however, in microalgae so far has not been found a correlation between the phenol content and DPPH, so this study shows the first evidence for a heterotrophic culture of *T. suecica*. Other authors differ from this relation, indicating that the variety of specific phenolic compounds in microalgae must be understood to which these correlation differences are attributed [48,53]. However, a synergistic effect among other compounds or substances could be involved in the antioxidant activity of microalgae, so future research would focus on correlating the increase in antioxidant activity in heterotrophic cultures with other variables involved in this type of condition.

2.5. Pigment Content of Autotrophic and Heterotrophic Biomass Cultures of T. suecica

The heterotrophic culture of *T. suecica* reduced chlorophyll and carotenoid levels to 1% and 12%, respectively ($p < 0.05$), with respect to that observed in autotrophy (Figure 1). Our results are in-line with those by Day and Tsavalos [33], who reported a reduction of chlorophyll levels to 1% and carotenes to 50% of *T. suecica* in heterotrophic culture, changing the cells from green to bright yellow, an adaptation caused by the absence of light and observed in higher plants [54].

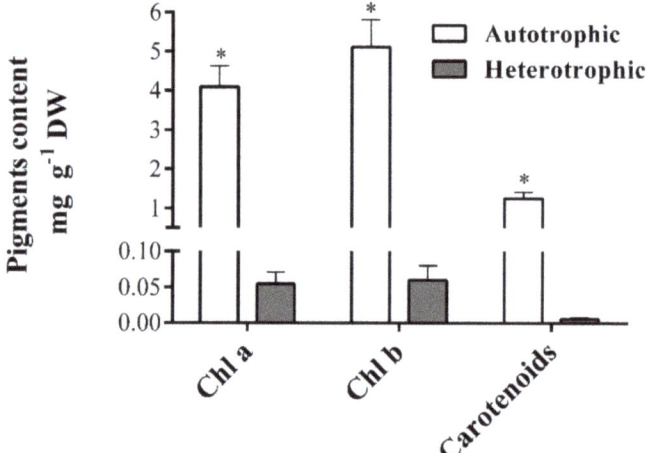

Figure 1. Pigment content extracted of the biomass from autotrophic and heterotrophic cultures of *Tetraselmis suecica* (mean ± SD; $n = 3$). Asterisks denote significant differences ($p < 0.05$, Student's *t*-test). DW: dry weight, Chl a and Chl b: chlorophyll-a and chlorophyll-b.

The reduction of photosynthetic and auxiliary pigments is related to the absence of light in heterotrophic cultures and to nitrogen depletion [41,55]. The stress generated by the changes in the trophic conditions and nutrients must be evaluated to identify potential microalgae that may produce some pigment of interest under dark conditions.

2.6. Production and Extraction of Exopolysaccharides (EPS) of Autotrophic and Heterotrophic Biomass Cultures of T. suecica

The maximum concentration of total and acid exopolysaccharides (EPS) extracted from the heterotrophic culture of *T. suecica* was 4.2 and 8 times higher, respectively, with respect to that obtained in the autotrophic culture ($p < 0.05$; Figure 2).

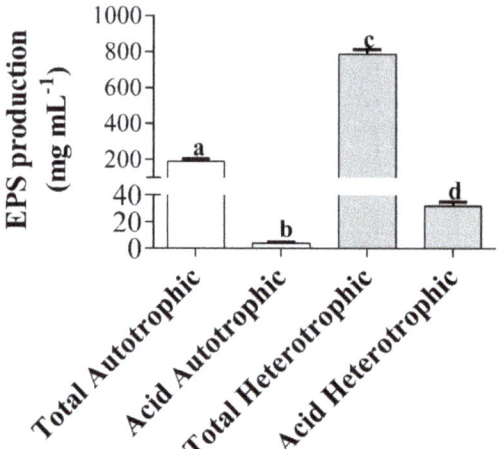

Figure 2. Total and acid exopolysaccharides (EPS) production from autotrophic and heterotrophic cultures of *T. suecica* (mean ± SD; $n = 3$). Different letters indicate significant differences (ANOVA, Tukey's test, $p < 0.05$).

The polysaccharide production for *T. suecica* has mainly focused on intracellular and cell wall polysaccharides [56]. Kashif et al. [57] showed that a treatment with 1-M NaOH in the biomass increased the yield and quality of polysaccharides of *Tetraselmis* sp. Dogra et al. [56] reported that the most efficient extraction of *T. suecica* polysaccharides was in the biomass treated with the Fenton reaction. This reaction increases the productivity of polysaccharides, because it generates oxidative stress to the microalgae biomass. Guzman-Murillo and Ascencio [26] extracted acid EPS from *T. suecica* and *Tetraselmis* sp. in which their maximum concentration was 409 mg L^{-1} and 1819 mg L^{-1}, respectively, values higher than those obtained in our study. The difference between our results and the ones previously cited [26] could be due to the different salinities used in the culture media. In our study, we used a salinity of 35 ‰, while the aforementioned authors used salinities of 3–6 ‰, which would indicate that *T. suecica* produces a greater amount of acidic EPS at low salinities. The osmotic adjustment and the regulation of the turgor pressure of the microalgae is affected by salinity, since, when it is low, the cellular ionic concentrations increase and their ionic relationships are constant. On the contrary, at salinities greater than 20‰, the ionic relationships are variable [58]. It is important to consider that these variations in ionic relationships play a fundamental role in the excretion of polysaccharides. Furthermore, these variations will also depend on the species and its adjustment mechanisms to osmotic stress. For example, in the case of *Botryococcus braunii*, the increase in salinity allowed a greater production of polysaccharides [59]. Therefore, the increase in EPS production in *T. suecica* will depend on the cultivation condition, abiotic factors such as salinity and optimization of EPS extraction methods.

2.7. Elemental Analysis of Exopolysaccharides (EPS) of Autotrophic and Heterotrophic Biomass Cultures of T. suecica

The acid EPS obtained from the heterotrophic culture of *T. suecica* showed the highest content of carbon and nitrogen ($p < 0.05$; Table 5), while acid and total EPS obtained from the autotrophic culture of *T. suecica* presented the lowest content of carbon and nitrogen, respectively. Although no sulfur was found in the autotrophic EPS, this element was present in the heterotrophic EPS, being statistically higher in acid EPS ($p < 0.05$). Total autotrophic EPS had the highest C/N ratio ($p < 0.05$), while the lowest C/N ratio was found in acid autotrophic EPS ($p < 0.05$). The EPS C/N ratio of microalgae, including *T. suecica*, has been poorly studied until now; therefore, the study of these relationships should be increased and specified. The sulfur content was only detected in the EPS of heterotrophic cultures. Within these, the acid EPS have a higher sulfur content than the total EPS ($p < 0.05$), mainly due to the fact that the extraction method is aimed exclusively at sulfated EPS.

Table 5. Total carbon (TC), total nitrogen (TN), ratio C/N and sulfur (S) (%) obtained in the total and acid polysaccharides extracted from autotrophic and heterotrophic cultures of *T. suecica*. The data represent the average ± standard deviation ($n = 3$). Different letters indicate significant differences among polysaccharide types (ANOVA, Tukey's test, $p < 0.05$).

Culture	Exopolysaccharide Type	% TC	% TN	C/N	% S
Autotrophic	Total	9.60 ± 0.10 [c]	0.53 ± 0.01 [d]	18.28 ± 0.17 [a]	0.00
Autotrophic	Acid	9.02 ± 0.08 [d]	0.71 ± 0.01 [b]	12.75 ± 0.10 [c]	0.00
Heterotrophic	Total	9.84 ± 0.07 [b]	0.66 ± 0.02 [c]	14.91 ± 0.10 [b]	0.33 ± 0.08 [b]
Heterotrophic	Acid	11.96 ± 0.09 [a]	0.80 ± 0.01 [a]	14.88 ± 0.12 [b]	3.47 ± 0.10 [a]

2.8. Antioxidant Activity of Exopolysaccharides (EPS) of Autotrophic and Heterotrophic Biomass Cultures of T. suecica

The total and acid heterotrophic EPS were 1.8 and 2.2 times higher than the autotrophic ones, respectively ($p < 0.05$; Figure 3).

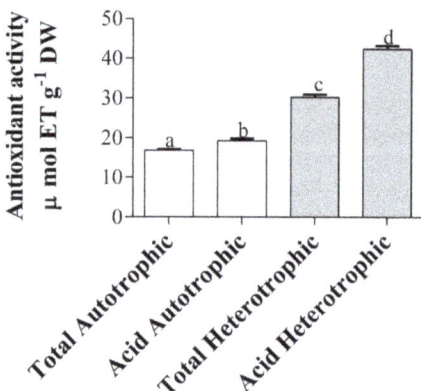

Figure 3. Antioxidant activity of total and acid exopolysaccharides from autotrophic and heterotrophic cultures of *T. suecica*. The antioxidant activity is expressed as micromoles of Trolox equivalents per gram of dry weight (μmol TE g^{-1} DW) (mean ± SD; $n = 3$). Different letters indicate significant differences (ANOVA, Tukey's test, $p < 0.05$).

The EPS from marine microalgae have shown the ability to protect oxidative stress, avoiding the accumulation of free radicals and reactive oxygen species (ROS) [28]. Dogra et al. [56] and Kashif et al. [57] reported the reducing capacity to eliminate radicals generated by ABTS, DPPH and FRAP methods for total EPS in the autotrophy of *Tetraselmis* sp. However, in the present study, it was only measured by the ABTS method, in which the total autotrophic EPS presented similar results. In the case of acid autotrophic EPS, and acid and total heterotrophic EPS, to the best of our knowledge, there are no previous references to this study, this being the first report of antioxidant activity for these types of *T. suecica* exopolysaccharides.

The antioxidant activity could be related to the percentage of galacturonic and glucuronic acids present in the constitution of the EPS of *T. suecica* (see Section 2.9). The heterotrophic EPS of *T. suecica* had sulfate in their constitution (Table 6), and, according to Mendiola et al. [30] and Sun et al. [60], the content of uronic acids and sulfate are related to an increase in the reducing capacity of free radicals [28]. The increase of these elements in the constitution of the heterotrophic EPS with respect to the autotrophic ones of *T. suecica* contributed to the increase of antioxidant activity. Possible phenols from ESPs were removed by precipitation with polyvinylpyrrolidone. It should be noted that it was not measured by the DPPH method, because its extraction is carried out in organic solvent, so the EPS immediately precipitated.

Table 6. Percentage of principal monosaccharides obtained in the total and acid polysaccharides extracted from autotrophic and heterotrophic cultures of *T. suecica*.

Monosaccharide	Autotrophic Total (%)	Autotrophic Acid (%)	Heterotrophic Total (%)	Heterotrophic Acid (%)
Arabinose	5.23	-	-	-
Ribose	0.83	0.65	1.22	0.33
Rhamnose	-	-	1.36	-
Fucose	-	-	0.38	0.35
Xylose	-	3.03	-	0.30
Mannose	6.64	1.57	36.15	34.49
Galacturonic acid	<0.10	2.93	2.45	2.95
Galactopyranoside	5.11	27.06	6.76	8.14
Galactose	25.27	9.96	3.00	2.93
Glucose	35.46	34.70	23.32	37.57
Glucuronic acid	21.47	20.10	25.36	22.94

2.9. Fourier-Transform Infrared Spectroscopy (FTIR) of Exopolysaccharides (EPS) of Autotrophic and Heterotrophic Biomass Cultures of T. suecica

FTIR spectroscopy of exopolysaccharides obtained from autotrophic and heterotrophic cultures of T. suecica showed the presence of various functional groups in all samples, such as hydroxyl or carbonyls groups (Figure 4). Although the autotrophic EPS of *T. suecica* did not present the sulfate group peak (Figure 4A,C), the heterotrophic ones did (Figure 4B,D). To the best of our knowledge, this is the first characterization of total and acid EPS extracted from autotrophic and heterotrophic cultures of *T. suecica*.

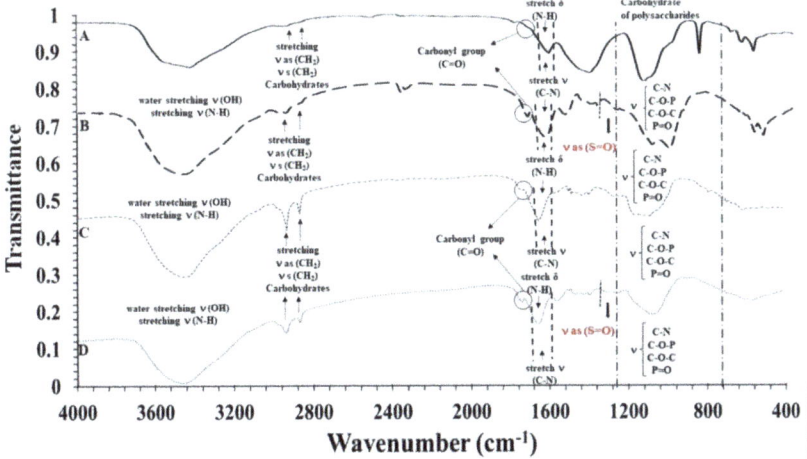

Figure 4. Fourier-transform infrared spectroscopy (FTIR) spectra of (**A**) total EPS obtained from the autotrophic culture of *T. suecica*, (**B**) total EPS obtained from the heterotrophic culture of *T. suecica*, (**C**) acid EPS obtained from the autotrophic culture of *T. suecica* and (**D**) acid EPS obtained from heterotrophic culture of *T. suecica*.

Different absorbance peaks were observed in the spectra of the autotrophic and heterotrophic EPS, indicating their functional groups (Figure 4). The strongest and widest signals were located between 3000 and 3500 cm^{-1}, which were attributed to the vibration of the -OH and -NH2 groups, followed by -CH2-methyl residues between 2800–2950 cm^{-1} characteristic of polysaccharides [61–63]. The peaks located between 1500 and 1700 cm^{-1} were due to the vibrations of the C=O groups and the stretching of C-N and the bending of NH [56,62,63]. The peak corresponding to the sulfate groups (S=O) was found between 1370–1240 cm^{-1} [64,65], which is characteristic of sulfated polysaccharides in marine microalgae [66]. The polysaccharides presented in the fingerprint zone from 1400 cm^{-1} to 700 cm^{-1}, presenting various stretching and deformations corresponding to the polysaccharides bonds (C-O-C, C-O-P, C-N and P=O) [67].

Dogra et al. [56] and Kashif et al. [57] carried out the FTIR analysis to the soluble fraction of polysaccharides of *Tetraselmis* sp. biomass in which they found the peak of 1650 cm^{-1} of vibrations of C=O in accordance with the present investigation. Furthermore, they found peaks between 1068–1079 cm^{-1} indicating -COOH with α helix amino acids (low molecular weight proteins) and 1049 cm^{-1} attributed to an aliphatic group with a possible increase in antioxidant activity. These two peaks were not shown in the present work. According to Meng et al. [68], the FTIR method is a validated spectroscopic method, which characterizes algae polysaccharides, determines variations of other primary metabolites and evaluates the physiology of microalgae. This characterization method could be used to temporarily observe the EPS excretion dynamics, and the comparison of the

2.10. Gas Chromatography—Mass Spectrometry (GC-MS) of Exopolysaccharides (EPS) of Autotrophic and Heterotrophic Biomass Cultures of T. suecica

In the GC-MS spectrum of total EPS extracted from the autotrophic culture of *T. suecica*, the highest peak corresponds to galactopyranoside with a retention time of 27.37 min, followed by glucose, galactose and glucuronic acid (Supplementary Figure S1). Other minor monosaccharides (mannose, arabinose and ribose) were identified.

In the GC-MS spectrum of acid EPS extracted from the autotrophic culture of *T. suecica*, the highest peak corresponds to glucose with a retention time of 28.93 min, followed by galactopyranoside, glucuronic acid and galactose (Supplementary Figure S2). Other minor monosaccharides were identified as xylose, galacturonic acid, mannose and ribose.

In the GC-MS spectrum of total EPS extracted from the heterotrophic culture of *T. suecica*, the highest peak corresponds to mannose with a retention time of 26.05 min, followed by glucose, glucuronic acid and rhamnose (Supplementary Figure S3). Other minor monosaccharides (galactose, galacturonic acid, ribose, and fucose) were identified.

In the GC-MS spectrum of acidic EPS extracted from the heterotrophic culture of *T. suecica*, the highest peak corresponds to mannose with a retention time of 26.06 min, followed by glucose, glucuronic acid and galactopyranoside (Supplementary Figure S4). Other minor monosaccharides were identified as galacturonic acid, galactose, fucose, ribose and xylose.

According to our revision, to the best of our knowledge, the monosaccharides of the EPS of *T. suecica* have not been previously characterized. However, intracellular and cell wall polysaccharides of *T. suecica* have been characterized as having 3-deoxy-D-manno-oct-2-ulosonic acid (Kdo) (54%), 3-deoxy-lyxo-2-heptulosaric acid (Dha) (17%), galacturonic acid (21%) and galactose (6%) by GC-MS [69]. For *Tetraselmis striata*, similar cell wall monosaccharides were described by NMR spectroscopy [70–72]. Dogra et al. [56] carried out the high-performance anion exchange chromatography with a pulsed amperometric detector (HPAEC-PAD) analysis to the soluble fraction of polysaccharides of *Tetraselmis* sp. biomass, in which they found that the KCTC 12432 BP strain contained a higher percentage of galactose and glucose in a molar ratio (11.1:8.2) and the strain KCTC 12236 BP showed the peaks of rhamnose, galactose, glucose, mannose and xylose. Therefore, the constitution of the EPS of *T. suecica* is different from the intracellular and cell wall polysaccharides. However, they have a similar monosaccharide composition with the soluble fraction of polysaccharides from *Tetraselmis* sp.

The EPS from autotrophic and heterotrophic cultures of *T. suecica* are composed in a higher percentage of glucose (23–37%), glucuronic acid (20–25%), mannose (2–36%), galactose (3–25%) and galactoryanoside (5–27%) and in lower percentages of galacturonic acid (0.1–3%); arabinose (5%); xylose (0.3–3%) and ribose, rhamnose and fucose (1%) (Table 6). Differences were found between the monosaccharide constitution of the EPS of autotrophic and heterotrophic cultures of this study. The highest percentage of mannose and fucose were the heterotrophic EPS, while the highest amounts of galactose and glucose were detected in autotrophic EPS. Xylose was present only in acid EPS from both culture conditions, while arabinose and rhamnose were found only in the total autotrophic and heterotrophic EPS.

According to Xiao and Zheng [73], the variations in EPS percentage are due to a nutritional stress of the culture conditions of origin of each one of them. These authors indicated that the differences and changes at the physiological level of the microalgae caused by different culture conditions make the microalgae adapt and biosynthesize polysaccharides according to the environmental conditions. Despite the percentages of monosaccharides presented for each EPS, the particular weight of each of the monosaccharides must be analyzed, representing the same high values of uronic acids in heterotrophy (galacturonic and glucuronic acids). According to de Jesus Raposo [28], polysaccharides with high contents of uronic acids present high bioactivity.

2.11. Cytotoxic Effects on Tumor Cells of Exopolysaccharides (EPS) of Autotrophic and Heterotrophic Biomass Cultures of T. suecica

The results obtained in this study showed that the EPS obtained from *T. suecica* in autotrophic and heterotrophic cultures have high cytotoxic effects on tumor cells (Figure 5). In the human leukemia cell line HL-60, inhibitory concentration (IC$_{50}$) of 36 µg mL^{-1} and 68 µg mL^{-1} were determined for acidic autotrophic and heterotrophic EPS, respectively, and IC$_{50}$ of 1784 µg mL^{-1} and 5183 µg mL^{-1} for total autotrophic and heterotrophic EPS, respectively (Figure 5A). In the breast cancer cell line (MCF-7), the acidic autotrophic and heterotrophic EPS showed IC$_{50}$ of 60 µg mL^{-1} and 141 µg mL^{-1}, respectively, while the total autotrophic and heterotrophic EPS showed lower effects with IC$_{50}$ of 9461 µg mL^{-1} and 9135 µg mL^{-1}, respectively (Figure 5B). In the case of the lung cancer cell line (NCI-H460), the acidic autotrophic and heterotrophic EPS showed high cytotoxic effects with IC$_{50}$ of 118 µg mL^{-1} and 110 µg mL^{-1}, respectively, whilst the total autotrophic and heterotrophic EPS had lower activity with IC$_{50}$ of 5160 µg mL^{-1} and 8000 µg mL^{-1}, respectively (Figure 5C).

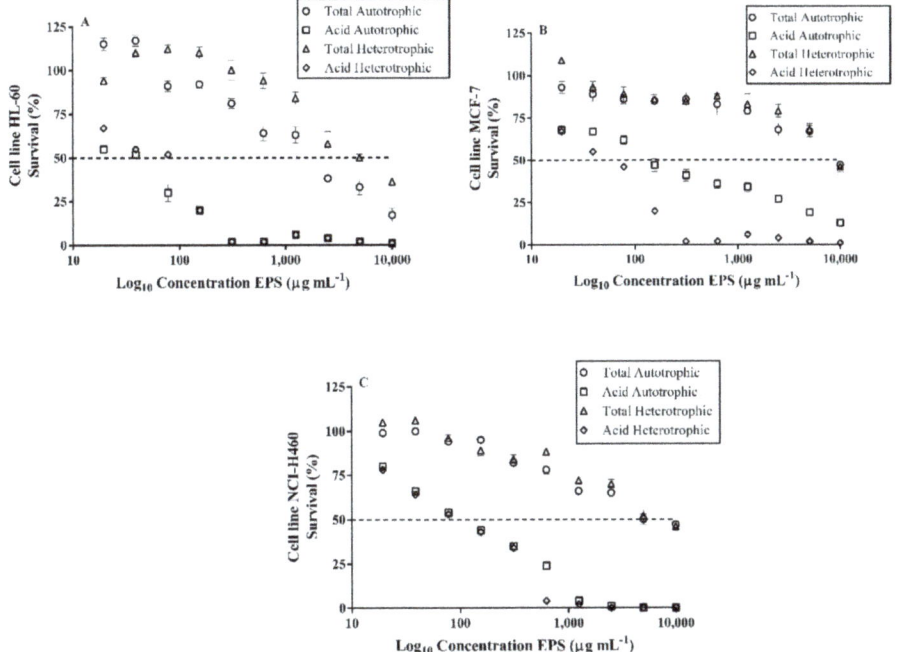

Figure 5. (**A**). Survival (%) of the human leukemia cell line (HL-60) exposed to different concentrations of EPS from *T. suecica*. (**B**). Survival (%) of the human breast cancer cell line (MCF-7) exposed to different concentrations of EPS from *T. suecica*. (**C**). Survival (%) of the human lung cancer cell line (NCI-H460) exposed to different concentrations of EPS from *T. suecica*.

This is the first evidence that EPS from *T. suecica* have cytotoxic effects on tumor cells. Previously, it has only been demonstrated that acidic EPS from *Tetraselmis* sp. inhibited the adhesion of *Helicobacter pylori* to HeLa S3 cells, indicating a possible prophylactic treatment in microbial infections, although in vivo experimental models are necessary [26]. Microalgae polysaccharides are interesting candidates for antitumor therapies. Polysaccharides from *Tribonema* sp. and *Phaedactylum tricornum* induced apoptosis in the liver cancer cell line (HepG2) [74,75]. Polysaccharides from *Artrosphira platensis* reduced cell proliferation in HepG2 and the breast cancer cell line (MCF-7) [76]. Other studies have described the antiproliferative activity of EPS from *Porphyridium cruentum* in the human cervical cancer cell line (HeLa) [77], MCF-7 cell line [78] and the inhibition of tumor growth Graffi myeloids [32]. Therefore, EPS from marine microalgae can be used as functional ingredients in foods or possible nutraceuticals to decrease the likelihood of tumor formation and development in the human body.

2.12. Cytotoxic of Exopolysaccharides (EPS) of Autotrophic and Heterotrophic Biomass Cultures of T. suecica

The autotrophic and heterotrophic total EPS did not reach the IC_{50} at the concentrations tested; therefore, they did not have a cytotoxic effect on the proliferation of the gingival fibroblast cell line (HGF-1) (Figure 6). However, the autotrophic and heterotrophic acid EPS showed cytotoxicity effects with IC_{50} of 165 µg mL^{-1} and 61 µg mL^{-1}, respectively (Figure 6). The elemental characteristic of cancer chemotherapeutics is that the compounds used do not affect the normal cell growth and have specific cytotoxicity [79]. Gingival fibroblast cell line (HGF-1) is a representative mammalian cell line that has been used for the investigation of anticancer activity [80]. Based on our results, the acids EPS showed high cytotoxicity; therefore, they are not suitable for therapeutic use. In contrast, the total EPS did not show cytotoxicity, so they could be a good candidate for anticancer investigation. However, it is important to deepen the studies and test other types of healthy cell lines.

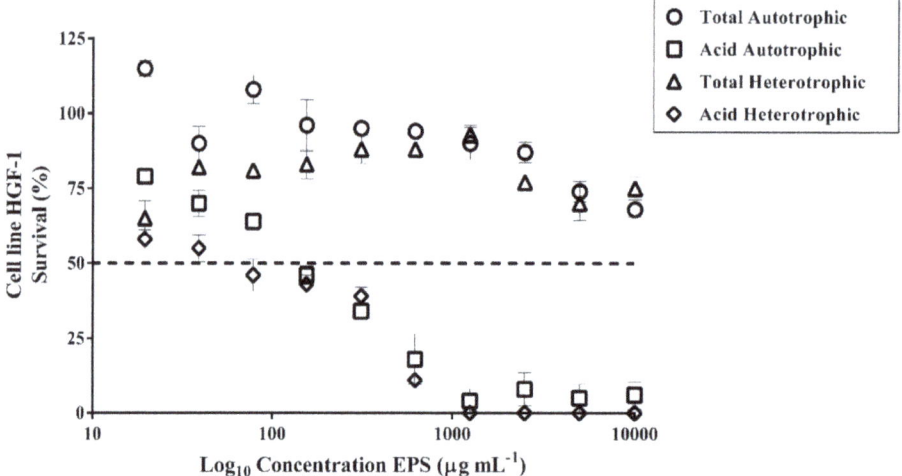

Figure 6. Survival (%) of the human gingival fibroblast cell line (HGF-1) exposed to different concentrations of EPS from *T. suecica*.

3. Materials and Methods

3.1. Biological Material

The strain used in this experiment, *T. suecica* (Chlorophyta), is part of the microalgae bank collection (strain code n° UMA-260920) of the Institute of Biotechnology and Blue Development (IBYDA) of Malaga University (Malaga, Andalucia, Spain).

3.2. Culture Conditions

3.2.1. Autotrophic Culture of *T. suecica*

The microalgae *T. suecica* was cultured in 100-mL glass photobioreactors with a diameter of 3.0 cm, with constant temperature (21 °C). The photoperiod was adjusted to 12 h of light (irradiance 165 µmol photons m^{-2} s^{-1}) and 12h of darkness (12:12) and was maintained in agitation with a constant air bubbling system in order to avoid microalgae sedimentation and achieving a homogeneous distribution of nutrients and irradiance in each cell. The culture was inoculated with a concentration of 6×10^5 cells mL^{-1} and adjusted to 35‰ salinity. The culture system was through a batch culture, with the addition of the culture medium F/2 [81]. The culture was volumetrically scaled to 10 L and was kept in a stationary phase. All the experiments were carried out in triplicate.

3.2.2. Heterotrophic Culture of *T. suecica*

The adaptation of an autotrophic to a heterotrophic culture of *T. suecica* was carried out in 100-mL glass photobioreactors with a diameter of 3.0 cm and constant temperature (21 °C). A batch culture system was started. The reduction of the photoperiod illumination time was progressive (light:dark) 12:12 (288 h), 8:16 (228 h), 4:20 (240 h), 3:21 (156 h), 2:22 (168 h) and 0:24. The culture medium used was F/2 supplemented with penicillin/streptomycin 0.1% *v/v*, with an optimal glucose dosage of 5 g L^{-1} in darkness condition. The culture was maintained with constant agitation by means of an air bubbling system, avoiding the sedimentation of the microalgae and achieving a homogeneous distribution of nutrients. Once the cultures were adapted to heterotrophy, they were volumetrically scaled to reach 2 L. All the experiments were carried out in triplicate.

3.3. Extraction Conditions

3.3.1. Biomass Extraction

In autotrophic and heterotrophic conditions, when the stationary phase was achieved, the culture was harvested by centrifugation at 3500 rpm for 8 min at 4 °C. The biomass was washed twice with distilled water to eliminate salts traces and was subsequently dried in an oven at 40 °C for 48 h. Once dried, it was stored at room temperature until further analyses.

3.3.2. Exopolysaccharides Extraction

Once the autotrophic and heterotrophic cultures reached the stationary phase, they were centrifuged at 3500 rpm for 8 min at 4 °C, and the supernatant was used for the extraction of total and acid EPS from *T. suecica*. Before extraction, phenols were removed by precipitation with polyvinylpyrrolidone (Sigma-Aldrich, St. Louis, MO, USA) and centrifugation 4500 rpm, 5 min, 4 °C. For this, total EPS were precipitated with the addition of ethanol (*v/v*) [82] and acid EPS with N-cetylpyridinium bromide (Cetavlon) (Sigma-Aldrich, St. Louis, MO, USA) 2% (*w/v*) for 24 h [83]. Then, the EPS were centrifuged at 4500 rpm for 5 min, 4 °C. The supernatant was discarded, and 10 mL of 4-M NaCl (Sigma-Aldrich, St. Louis, MO, USA) was added. This mix was stirred until completely dissolved. Once cooled, ethanol was placed in a ratio (*v/v*) and kept at 4 °C for 24 h. After centrifugation at 4500 rpm, 5 min, 4 °C, the pellet containing the polysaccharides and salts was placed on a dialysis membrane (Sigma-Aldrich, St. Louis, MO, USA) in a 0.5-M NaCl solution overnight at 4 °C. Then, the dialyzed EPS was centrifuged at 4500 rpm for 5 min, 4 °C, and washed with absolute ethanol. Finally, acid and total EPS from both culture conditions (per triplicate, $n = 3$) were stored at −80 °C and subsequently freeze-dried at −50 °C. The EPS were quantified on an analytical balance, and the maximum concentrations obtained in the autotrophic and heterotrophic cultures were compared according to the culture volume and cell density.

3.4. Population Parameters (Cell Density, Cell Concentration, Specific Growth Rate, Biovolume and Cell Volume)

Cell concentration was calculated according to Equation 1 [84]:

$$Cell\ concentration = \left(\frac{W_1 - W_0}{Volume}\right) \quad (1)$$

where W_1 and W_0 are the differences in total weight of cells g L^{-1} at volume filtration.

Through cell quantification in a 100-μm cuvette (Beckman Coulter™ AccuComp Z2, Indianapolis, IN, USA), at a pre-established dilution of 1/20, the specific growth rate μ (day^{-1}) and the daily doubling of biomass was calculated, and the results were shown as the sum of these with the algorithm of Arredondo and Voltolina [84], summarized in Equation (2):

$$\mu = \frac{\ln(N_2 - N_1)}{t_2 - t_1} \quad (2)$$

where N_2 and N_1 are the density of cells mL^{-1} at times t_2 and t_1, respectively.

The biovolume was calculated from the mean of the population (μm^3 cell^{-1}) provided by cell quantification and the value of the cell density (cell mL^{-1}) to obtain its final value in μm^3 mL^{-1}.

3.5. Total Carbon (C), Hydrogen (H), Nitrogen (N) and Sulfur (S) of Dry Biomass and Exopolysaccharides

Total carbon (C), nitrogen (N) and sulfur (S) were determined from dry biomass and the extracted polysaccharides using the total combustion technique used in the LECO TruSppec Micro CHNSO-Elemental Analyzer (St. Joseph, MI, USA). This technique is based on the complete and instantaneous oxidation of the sample by pure combustion with controlled oxygen at a temperature of up to 1050 °C (C, H, N and S) and pyrolysis at 1300 °C (O) for decomposition of O as CO and oxidation to CO_2. The resulting combustion products, CO_2, H_2O, SO_2 and N_2 are subsequently quantified by selective IR Pleabsorption detector (C, H and S) and TCD (N) differential thermoconductivity sensor. The result of each element (C, H, N and S) is expressed in % with respect to the weight of the sample.

3.6. Biochemical Composition of Autotrophic and Heterotrophic Biomass Cultures of T. suecica

For the biochemical composition ($n = 3$), total proteins were calculated from the elemental N determination using the N-protein conversion factor of 4.80 reported by Lourenço et al. [85]; lipids were extracted according to the Folch method [86] and carbohydrates according to the phenol-sulfuric procedure [87]. Moisture and ash levels were determined gravimetrically by drying in an oven at 105 °C and after incineration in a muffle furnace at 550 °C, respectively, until constant weight.

3.7. Determination of Phenolic Compounds

Quantification of phenolic compounds was performed according to the Folin-Ciocalteu method [88]. Reaction was performed by adding 20 mg of biomass and placed in an Eppendorf with 1 mL of 80% methanol (Sigma-Aldrich, St. Louis, MO, USA). The solution was stirred and incubated at 4 °C in darkness for 12 to 24 h. Following this, the solution was centrifuged at 3500 rpm for 10 min, 4 °C. Then, 100 μL of the extract, 700 μL of distilled water, 150 μL of 20% anhydrous sodium carbonate (Na_2CO_3) (Sigma-Aldrich, St. Louis, MO, USA) and 50 μL of the Folin-Ciocalteu reagent (Sigma-Aldrich, St. Louis, MO, USA) were mixed by stirring and incubated at 4 °C in darkness for 2 h. The absorbance was measured at 760 nm using a UV–visible spectrophotometer (SHIMADZU UV MINI-1240, Duisburg, Germany). The blank included all reagents, except the extract that was replaced by 80% methanol. Phenolic contents were determined by constructing a standard curve using different phloroglucinol (Sigma-Aldrich, St. Louis, MO, USA) concentrations. Results were expressed in the mg equivalent of phloroglucinol per g of algal dry weight (DW).

3.8. Determination of Pigments

For chlorophyll a, chlorophyll b and total carotenoid quantification, an acetone 90% extract was done with 5 mg of freeze-dried biomass in 1 mL of solvent. The extract was sonicated for 3 min and remained 24 h in darkness at 4 °C. Chlorophyll a was determined according to Equation (3) [89], chlorophyll b was determined according to Equation 4 [90] and total carotenoids were determined according to Equation (5) [91].

$$[(11.8668 \times A_{664}) - (-1.7858 \times A_{647})] \tag{3}$$

$$[(18.9775 \times A_{647}) - (-4.8950 \times A_{664})] \tag{4}$$

$$[(A_{480} \times 4.0)] \tag{5}$$

where A_{664}, A_{647} and A_{480} are the measured absorbance at 667, 647 and 480 nm, respectively.

3.9. Lipopolysaccharides (LPS) Contamination Assay

The presence of lipopolysaccharides (LPS) in the EPS fractions isolated from *T. suecica* was evaluated using the *Limulus* amebocyte lysate (LAL) assay kit (Endosafe®-PTS, Charles River Laboratories, Charleston, SC, USA). In brief, 25 µL of the EPS solution (concentration 50 µg mL^{-1}) in distilled water was loaded into each of the four channels of the cartridge. The reader automatically mixed the sample with the LAL reagent in two channels. Additionally, the LAL reagent was mixed with the positive control in the other two channels. These samples were used as the control. Afterward, all samples were incubated and combined with the chromogenic substrate. After mixing, the optical density of the four channels was measured and compared with an internal standard curve. The amount of endotoxin in the sample was expressed as endotoxin units (EU) mL^{-1}.

3.10. Antioxidant Capacity

3.10.1. ABTS Assay Scavenging of Free Radical in Exopolysaccharides and Biomass

The ability of the polysaccharides to scavenge the free radicals was evaluated using an ABTS assay according to Re et al. [92], with few modifications. ABTS radical cation was produced through the reaction with the 2,2′-azino-bis (3-ethylbenzothiazoline-6-sulphonic acid) (ABTS) 7-mM solution with 2.45-mM potassium persulfate for 16h in the dark at 4 °C. After incubation, the well-mixed solution was diluted to an absorbance of 0.7 at 727 nm with the deionized water. For biomass and EPS, 10 mg were weighted, and 1 mL of phosphate buffer was added, mechanically disrupted and centrifuged at 4 °C for 5 min at 3500 rpm. A total of 50 µL of these samples (supernatant in case of biomass) were mixed with 940 µL of phosphate buffer and 10 µL of ABTS solution. The resulting mixture was measured with a spectrophotometer at 727 nm. ABTS radical scavenging capacity was calculated according to Equation (6) [93]:

$$AA\% = (Abs_0 - Abs_1 / Abs_0) \times 100 \tag{6}$$

where Abs_0 is the absorbance of the ABTS radical in phosphate buffer at time 0, and Abs_1 is the absorbance of the ABTS radical solution mixed with the sample after 8 min. A calibration curve was performed with different concentrations of Trolox® (0 to 5 µg mL^{-1}) from a stock of Trolox® 2.5 mM. The % inhibition was determined by interpolation of the absorbance values in the Trolox standard curve fitted to the equation of a linear regression line (y = 13.593x + 0.8717; R^2 = 0.99). All determinations were performed in triplicate (n = 3).

3.10.2. DPPH Free-Radical Method in Biomass from *T. suecica*

Radical scavenging and antioxidant activities of the extracts of biomass were assessed by the 2,2-diphenyl-1-picrylhydrazyl (DPPH) free-radical method by Brand-Williams et al. [94]. To obtain the extracts from the biomass, 10 mg of the sample was weighted, and 1 mL of 80% methanol was added, homogenized by mechanical disruption, and left for 16 h in the dark at 4 °C. After incubation, samples were centrifuged at 4 °C for 5 min at 3500 rpm. Aliquots of 200 µL of the supernatant samples were added to 90 µL of instantly prepared DPPH solution (0.358 mM) and 910 µL 80% methanol.

The samples were incubated in the dark for 30 min at room temperature, and the absorbance (abs) was read at 517 nm against 80% methanol as blank. The absorbance was then transformed into a percentage of inhibition versus 80% methanol. The percentage of the antioxidant activity was calculated according to Equation (7) [93].

$$AA\% = [(Abs_0 - Abs_1) Abs_0] \times 100 \tag{7}$$

where Abs_0 is absorbance at time zero, and Abs_1 is absorbance at the end of the reaction (30 min) at 517 nm. A calibration curve was performed with different concentrations of Trolox® (0 to 7.5 µg mL^{-1}) from a stock of Trolox® 2.5 mM. The % inhibition was determined by interpolation of the absorbance values in the Trolox standard curve fitted to the equation of a linear regression line (y = 13.593x + 0.8717; R^2 = 0.99). All determinations were performed in triplicate (n = 3).

3.11. Fourier-Transform Infrared Spectroscopy (FTIR)

Fourier-transform infrared (FTIR) spectra of the polysaccharides from *T. suecica* were obtained by using self-supporting pressed discs of 13 mm in diameter of a mixture of polysaccharides and KBr (1% *w/w*) with a hydrostatic press at a force of 15.0 tcm^{-2} for 2 min. The FTIR spectra were obtained with a Thermo Nicolet Avatar 360 IR spectrophotometer (Thermo Electron Inc., Franklin, MA, USA) having a resolution of 4 cm^{-1} with a deuterated triglycine sulfate (DTGS) detector and using Omnic^{TM} 7.2 software (bandwidth 50 cm^{-1} and enhancement factor 2.6) in the 400–4000 cm^{-1} region. Baseline adjustment was performed using the Thermo Nicolet OMNIC software to flatten the baseline of each spectrum. The OMNIC correlation algorithm was used to compare sample spectra with those of the spectral library (Thermo Fisher Scientific, San Jose, CA, USA).

3.12. Gas chromatography–Mass Spectrometry (GC-MS)

3.12.1. Hydrolysis and Derivatization of EPS

Polysaccharides samples (2 mg) and monosaccharides standards were treated with the same procedure. First, 100 µL of the standard stock solution of 1 mg mL^{-1} of each monosaccharide was dried under nitrogen gas flow. Second, the samples of polysaccharides, and a mixture containing the standard monosaccharides included in the IS (Internal Standard), were methanolized in 2-mL methanol/3-M HCl at 80 °C during 24 h. The monosaccharides glucose, galactose, rhamnose, fructose, mannose, xylose, apiose and myo-inositol (Internal Standard, IS), as well as pyridine, hexane and methanol/3-M HCl solution, were purchased from Sigma-Aldrich. Then, the saccharides were washed with methanol and dried under nitrogen gas flow. Third, the trimethylsilyl reaction was accomplished with 200 µL of Tri-Sil HTP (Thermo Fisher Scientific, Franklin, MA, USA). Each vial with the sample was heated at 80 °C for 1 h. The derivatized sample was cooled to a room temperature and dried under a steam of nitrogen. Forth, the dry residue was extracted with hexane (2 mL) and centrifuged. Finally, the hexane solution containing silylated monosaccharides was concentrated and reconstituted in hexane (200 µL), filtered and transferred to a GC-MS autosampler vial. Sample preparation and analyses were performed in triplicate.

3.12.2. Gas Chromatography/Mass Spectrometry (GC-MS) Analysis

GC/MS analyses were carried out using a gas chromatograph Trace GC (Thermo Fisher Scientific, Franklin, MA, USA), an autosampler Triplus RSH (Thermo Fisher Scientific, Franklin, MA, USA) and a DSQ mass spectrometer quadrupole (Thermo Fisher Scientific, Franklin, MA, USA). The GC column was set ZB-5 Zebron, Phenomenex (5% phenyl and 95% dimethylpolysiloxane), 30-m (length) × 0.25-mm (I.D) × 0.25-µm film thickness. Injection volume was 1 µL in split mode, with a split ratio of 40. Helium was used as the carrier gas with a flow rate of 1.2 mL min^{-1}. The injector was set at 250 °C in split mode. The initial oven temperature was 80 °C for 2 min, then ramped from 10 °C min^{-1} to 180 °C, followed by ramping from 5 °C min^{-1} to 250 °C, remaining constant for 2 min. The electron impact ionization (EI) mode of the mass spectrometer was set at 70 eV. Monitored in full scan mode with mass range 50-650 *m/z* with interface temperature 250 °C and ionization source temperature of 230 °C. The identification of monosaccharides in polysaccharide samples was carried out by comparing retention time and mass spectra of monosaccharide standards, previously analyzed under identical conditions (glucose, galactose, mannose, arabinose, xylose, rhamnose, ribose, fucose, galacturonic acid and glucuronic acid). The compounds were identified by comparing the mass spectra with those in the National Institute of Standards and Technology (NIST 2014) library.

3.13. Cell Line Cultures

In this study, four cell lines were used: three of them tumoral, such as the human breast adenocarcinoma cell line (MCF-7, ATCC, Manassas, VA, USA), human leukemia cell line (HL-60 ATCC), human lung cancer cell line (NCI-H460, ATCC) and an immortalized human gingival fibroblast-1 cell line HGF-1 (ATCC CRL-2014). MCF-7 and HGF-1 cell lines were routinely cultured in Dulbecco's modified Eagle's medium (DMEM) (Biowest, Barcelona, Spain) supplemented with 10% fetal bovine serum (Biowest, Barcelona, Spain), 1% penicillin-streptomycin solution 100X and 0.5% of amphotericin B (Biowest, Barcelona, Spain), while NCI-H460 cells were cultured in Roswell Park Memorial Institute (RPMI-1640) medium (Biowest, Barcelona, Spain) supplemented with 10% fetal bovine serum, 1% penicillin-streptomycin solution 100X and 0.5% of amphotericin B, and HL-60 cells were cultured in RPMI-1640 medium (Biowest, Barcelona, Spain) supplemented with 20% fetal bovine serum, 1% penicillin-streptomycin solution 100X and 0.5% of amphotericin B (Biowest, Barcelona, Spain). Cells were maintained sub-confluent at 37 °C in humidified air containing 5% CO_2. Cultured cells were collected by gentle scraping when confluence was reached 75% in the case of the MCF-7, HFG-1 and NCI-H460, as they are adherent cells. The scrapping of HL-60 cells was not performed, because these are cells in suspension. So, they were collected by centrifugation at 1500 rpm for 5 min.

3.14. Cytotoxic Effects on Tumor Cells Assay

For cytotoxic effects on the tumor cells assay, HL-60, MCF-7 and NCI-H460 cell lines were incubated at 2×10^4, 8×10^3 and 8×10^3 cell lines per well, respectively in the presence of different concentrations ($19 - 1 \times 10^4$ µg mL^{-1}) of EPS. The experiment was conducted individually with each cell line in a 96-well microplate (Sarstedt, Nümbrecht, Germany) for 72 h. The incubation conditions were as follows: temperature 37 °C, 5% CO_2 and a humid atmosphere. As a control, the same cell lines were used without treatment. The proliferation of these cell lines was estimated by the MTT (Sigma-Aldrich, St. Louis, MO, USA) (3-(4,5-dimethylthiazol-2-yl)-2,5-diphenyltetrazolium bromide) assay [31]. Briefly, a volume of 10 µL of the MTT solution (5 mg mL^{-1} in phosphate-buffered saline) was added to each well. The microplates were incubated at 37 °C for 4 h. The yellow tetrazolium salt of MTT was reduced by mitochondrial dehydrogenases of metabolically active viable cells to form insoluble purple formazan crystals. Formazan was dissolved by the addition of sulfated–isopropanol (150 µL of 0.04-N HCl–2 propanol) and measured spectrophotometrically at 550 nm (Micro Plate Reader 2001, Whittaker Bioproducts, Promega, Wisconsin, USA). The relative cell viability was expressed as the mean percentage of viable cells compared with untreated cells. Four samples for each tested concentration were included in each experiment. Measurements were carried out in triplicate independent experiments.

3.15. Cytotoxicity Assay in Healthy Cell Line

For the cytotoxicity assay, HGF-1 cells were incubated at 1.5×10^4 cells per wells in the presence of different concentration of EPS ($19-1 \times 10^4$ µg mL^{-1}) in a 96-well microplate (Sarstedt, Nümbrecht, Germany) for 72 h. The incubation conditions were as follows: temperature 37 °C, 5% CO_2 and a humid atmosphere. Cells proliferation was estimated by the MTT (Sigma-Aldrich, St. Louis, MO, USA) (3-(4,5-dimethylthiazol-2-yl)-2,5-diphenyltetrazolium bromide) assay [31], as explained above.

3.16. Statistical Analysis

For the statistical analysis of the experimental results, the STATISTICA software (V.7; Tulsa, OK, USA) was used. All values were expressed as mean ± standard deviations (SD). The one-way analysis of variance (ANOVA) was used to determine the differences between the EPS production, elemental analysis of EPS and antioxidant activity of EPS. When significant differences in the ANOVA were found, the post-hoc Tukey test was performed to identify the difference between the treatments. The Student's *t*-test was used to determine significant differences between the cultures in all population parameters, biochemical composition, C/N ratio, phenolic compounds, antioxidant activity and pigments. Homogeneity of variance was checked using the Cochran test and by visual inspection of the residues [95]. The correlations of the data obtained were calculated using Pearson's correlation analysis. Statistical significance of mean differences was considered to be attained with $p < 0.05$.

4. Conclusions

We determined that the heterotrophic conditions have several advantages over the autotrophic, such as improving the biochemical composition; enhancing the accumulation of proteins, lipids and carbohydrates and increasing the yield of exopolysaccharides (EPS). The antioxidant activity of the heterotrophic crop was higher with respect to the autotrophic crop, as well as for the algal biomass and EPS. In addition, to the best of our knowledge, this is the first time that autotrophic and heterotrophic EPS of *T. suecica* proved to have cytotoxic effects on HL-60, MCF-7 and NCI-H460 tumor cells. Therefore, they could offer greater benefits as possible natural nutraceuticals for the pharmaceutical industry. More studies are necessary to identify the specific bioactive fractions of each EPS.

Supplementary Materials: The following are available online at http://www.mdpi.com/1660-3397/18/11/534/s1: Figure S1–S4: Gas chromatography-mass spectrometry (GC-MS) analysis. Table S1: Pearson correlation between variables from the heterotrophic culture of *T. suecica* ($n = 3$).

Author Contributions: Conceptualization, G.P.-R., E.U.-T. and R.T.A-D.; methodology, G.P.-T. and V.C.-A.; software, G.P.-R. and J.G.-M.; validation, G.P.-R., J.G.-.M. and R.T.A-D.; investigation, G.P.-R.; data curation, G.P.-R., J.G.-M. and V.C-.A.; writing—original draft preparation, G.P.-R., J.G.-M. and V.C-.A.; writing—review and editing, G.P.-R., J.G.-M., E.U.-T. and R.T. A.-D.; visualization, G.P.-R., E.U.-T. and R.T.A.-D.; project administration, G.P.-R. and funding acquisition, G.P.-R. All authors have read and agreed to the published version of the manuscript.

Funding: This research was funded by the ANID-PFCHA National Doctoral Scholarship, 2018-N° 21180059 and FCAC N° 057/2019-UCN.

Acknowledgments: We want to express our gratitude to the Photobiology and Biotechnology of Aquatic Organisms (FYBOA) research group (RNM-295) for their technical support. We also want to thank the Cell Culture Unit of the SCAI (Central Research Support Service) of the University of Malaga for the technical assistance in the use of the laboratory. We also want to thank the Primary Production Laboratory of the Universidad Catolica del Norte for the use of the laboratory for the development of microalgal cultures.

Conflicts of Interest: The authors declare no conflict of interest.

References

1. Brennan, L.; Owende, P. Biofuels from microalgae—A review of technologies for production, processing, and extractions of biofuels and co-products. *Renew. Sustain. Energy Rev.* **2010**, *14*, 557–577. [CrossRef]
2. Vásquez-Piñeros, M.A.; Rondón-Barragan, I.S.; Eslava-Mocha, P.R.; Marina, B. Inmunoestimulantes en teleosteos: Probióticos, β-glucanos y LPS. *Orinoquia* **2012**, *16*, 46–62. [CrossRef]
3. Huang, G.; Chen, F.; Wei, D.; Zhang, X.; Chen, G. Biodiesel production by microalgal biotechnology. *Appl. Energy* **2010**, *87*, 38–46. [CrossRef]
4. Acién, F.; Gómez-Serrano, C.; Morales-Amaral, M.; Fernández-Sevilla, J.; Molina-Grima, E. Wastewater treatment using microalgae: How realistic a contribution might it be to significant urban wastewater treatment? *Appl. Microbiol. Biotechnol.* **2016**, *100*, 9013–9022. [CrossRef] [PubMed]
5. Pérez-García, O.; Escalante, F.M.E.; De-Bashan, L.E.; Bashan, Y. Heterotrophic cultures of microalgae: Metabolism and potential products. *Water Res.* **2011**, *45*, 11–36. [CrossRef] [PubMed]

6. Morales-Sánchez, D.; Martinez-Rodriguez, O.A.; Kyndt, J.; Martinez, A. Heterotrophic growth of microalgae: Metabolic aspects. *World J. Microbiol. Biotechnol.* **2015**, *31*, 1–9. [CrossRef] [PubMed]
7. Morales-Sánchez, D.; Martinez-Rodriguez, O.A.; Martinez, A. Heterotrophic cultivation of microalgae: Production of metabolites of commercial interest. *J. Chem. Technol. Biotechnol.* **2017**, *92*, 925–936. [CrossRef]
8. Borowitzka, M.A. Algal Physiology and Large-Scale Outdoor Cultures of Microalgae. In *The Physiology of Microalgae: Developments in Applied Phycology*; Borowitzka, M., Beardall, M., Rave, J., Eds.; Springer: Cham, Switzerland, 2016; Volume 6, pp. 601–652.
9. Velea, S.; Oancea, F.; Fischer, F. Heterotrophic and mixotrophic microalgae cultivation. In *Microalgae-Based Biofuels and Bioproducts*; Gonzalez-Fernandez, C., Muñoz, R., Eds.; Woodhead Publishing Elsevier: Kindlington, UK, 2017; pp. 45–65.
10. Barros, A.; Pereira, H.; Campos, J.; Marques, A.; Varela, J.; Silva, J. Heterotrophy as a tool to overcome the long and costly autotrophic scale-up process for large scale production of microalgae. *Sci. Rep.* **2019**, *9*, 1–7. [CrossRef]
11. Xu, H.; Miao, X.; Wu, Q. High quality biodiesel production from a microalga *Chlorella protothecoides* by heterotrophic growth in fermenters. *J. Biotechnol.* **2006**, *126*, 499–507. [CrossRef]
12. Azma, M.; Shamzi Mohamed, M.; Mohamad, R.; Abdul Rahim, R.; Ariff, A.B. Improvement of medium composition for heterotrophic cultivation of green microalgae, *Tetraselmis suecica*, using response surface methodology. *Biochem. Eng. J.* **2011**, *53*, 187–195. [CrossRef]
13. Leyva, L.A.; Bashan, Y.; Mendoza, A.; de-Bashan, L.E. Accumulation fatty acids of in *Chlorella vulgaris* under heterotrophic conditions in relation to activity of acetyl-CoA carboxylase, temperature, and co-immobilization with *Azospirillum brasilense*. *Naturwissenschaften* **2014**, *101*, 819–830. [CrossRef] [PubMed]
14. Gladue, R.M.; Maxey, J.E. Microalgal feeds for aquaculture. *J. Appl. Phycol.* **1994**, *6*, 131–141. [CrossRef]
15. Choix, F.J.; De-Bashan, L.E.; Bashan, Y. Enhanced accumulation of starch and total carbohydrates in alginate-immobilized *Chlorella* spp. induced by *Azospirillum brasilense*: II. Heterotrophic conditions. *Enzym. Microb. Technol.* **2012**, *51*, 300–309. [CrossRef]
16. El-Sheekh, M.M.; Bedaiwy, M.Y.; Osman, M.E.; Ismail, M.M. Mixotrophic and heterotrophic growth of some microalgae using extract of fungal-treated wheat bran. *Int. J. Recycl. Org. Waste Agric.* **2012**, *1*, 1–9. [CrossRef]
17. Sloth, J.K.; Wiebe, M.G.; Eriksen, N.T. Accumulation of phycocyanin in heterotrophic and mixotrophic cultures of the acidophilic red alga *Galdieria sulphuraria*. *Enzym. Microb. Technol.* **2006**, *38*, 168–175. [CrossRef]
18. Graverholt, O.S.; Eriksen, N.T. Heterotrophic high-cell-density fed-batch and continuous-flow cultures of *Galdieria sulphuraria* and production of phycocyanin. *Biotechnol. Bioprocess. Eng.* **2007**, *77*, 69–75. [CrossRef] [PubMed]
19. Wu, Z.Y.; Shi, C.L.; Shi, X.M. Modeling of lutein production by heterotrophic *Chlorella* in batch and fed-batch cultures. *World J. Microbiol. Biotechnol.* **2007**, *23*, 1233–1238. [CrossRef]
20. Day, J.; Edwards, A.; Rodgers, G. Development of an industrial-scale process for the heterotrophic production of a microalgal mollusc feed. *Bioresour. Technol.* **1991**, *38*, 245–249. [CrossRef]
21. Azma, M.; Mohamad, R.; Rahim, R.A.; Ariff, A.B. Improved Protocol for the Preparation of *Tetraselmis suecica* Axenic Culture and Adaptation to Heterotrophic Cultivation. *Open Biotechnol. J.* **2010**, *4*, 36–46. [CrossRef]
22. Austin, B.; Day, J.G. Inhibition of prawn pathogenic *Vibrio* spp. by a commercial spray-dried preparation of *Tetraselmis suecica*. *Aquaculture* **1990**, *90*, 389–392. [CrossRef]
23. Austin, B.; Baudet, E.; Stobie, M. Inhibition of bacterial fish pathogens by *Tetraselmis suecica*. *J. Fish. Dis.* **1992**, *15*, 55–61. [CrossRef]
24. Irianto, A.; Austin, B. Probiotics in aquaculture. *J. Fish. Dis.* **2002**, *25*, 633–642. [CrossRef]
25. Carballo-Cárdenas, E.C.; Tuan, M.; Janssen, M.; Wijffels, R.H. Vitamin E (a-tocopherol) production by the marine microalgae *Dunaliella tertiolecta* and *Tetraselmis suecica* in batch cultivation. *Biomol. Eng.* **2003**, *20*, 139–147. [CrossRef]
26. Guzman-Murillo, M.; Ascencio, F. Anti-adhesive activity of sulphated exopolysaccharides of microalgae on attachment of red sore disease-associated bacteria and *Helicobacter pylori* to tissue culture cells. *Lett. Appl. Microbiol.* **2000**, *30*, 473–478. [CrossRef]
27. Pontis, H.G. Case Study: Polysaccharides. In *Methods for Analysis of Carbohydrate Metabolism in Photosynthetic Organisms: Plants, Green Algae and Cyanobacteria*; Pontis, H., Ed.; Elsevier Academic Press: Cambridge, MA, USA, 2016; pp. 137–149.

28. De Jesus Raposo, M.F.; de Morais, A.M.; de Morais, R.M. Bioactivity and Applications of Polysaccharides from Marine Microalgae. In *Polysaccharides*; Ramawat, K., Mérillon, J., Eds.; Springer: Cham, Switzerland, 2015; pp. 1683–1727.
29. Rupérez, P.; Ahrazem, O.; Leal, J.A. Potential antioxidant capacity of sulfated polysaccharides from the edible marine brown seaweed *Fucus vesiculosus*. *J. Agric. Food Chem.* **2002**, *50*, 840–845. [CrossRef]
30. Mendiola, J.A.; Jaime, L.; Santoyo, S.; Reglero, G.; Cifuentes, A.; Ibañez, E.; Señoráns, F.J. Screening of functional compounds in supercritical fluid extracts from *Spirulina platensis*. *Food Chem.* **2007**, *102*, 1357–1367. [CrossRef]
31. Abdala Díaz, R.T.; Casas Arrojo, V.; Arrojo Agudo, M.A.; Cárdenas, C.; Dobretsov, S.; Figueroa, F.L. Immunomodulatory and Antioxidant Activities of Sulfated Polysaccharides from *Laminaria ochroleuca*, *Porphyra umbilicalis*, and *Gelidium corneum*. *Mar. Biotechnol.* **2019**, *21*, 577–587. [CrossRef] [PubMed]
32. Gardeva, E.; Toshkova, R.; Minkova, K.; Gigova, L. Cancer Protective Action of Polysaccharide, Derived from Red Microalga *Porphyridium cruentum*-A Biological Background. *Biotechnol. Biotechnol Equip.* **2009**, *23*, 783–787. [CrossRef]
33. Day, J.; Tsavalos, A. An investigation of the heterotrophic culture of the green alga *Tetraselmis*. *J. Appl. Phycol.* **1996**, *8*, 73–77. [CrossRef]
34. Walne, P. Studies on food value of nineteen genera of algae to juvenile bivalvies of the genera *Ostrea*. *Fish. Invest. Lond. Ser.* **1970**, 1–62.
35. Razaghi, A.; Godhe, A.; Albers, E. Effects of nitrogen on growth and carbohydrate formation in *Porphyridium cruentum*. *Cent. Eur. J. Biol* **2014**, *9*, 156–162. [CrossRef]
36. Cheng, Y.; Zhou, W.; Gao, C.; Lan, K.; Gao, Y.; Wu, Q. Biodiesel production from Jerusalem artichoke (*Helianthus tuberosus* L.) tuber by heterotrophic microalgae *Chlorella protothecoides*. *J. Chem. Technol. Biotechnol.* **2009**, *84*, 777–781. [CrossRef]
37. Cid, A.; Abalde, J.; Herrero, C. Crecimiento y composición bioquímica de la microalga marina *Tetraselmis suecica* en cultivos mixotróficos con distintos azúcares y aminoácidos. *Cah. Biol. Mar.* **1992**, *33*, 169–178.
38. Canelli, G.; Neutsch, L.; Carpine, R.; Tevere, S.; Giuffrida, F.; Rohfritsch, Z.; Dionisi, F.; Bolten, C.; Mathys, A. *Chlorella vulgaris* in a heterotrophic bioprocess: Study of the lipid bioaccessibility and oxidative stability. *Algal Res.* **2020**, *45*, 101754. [CrossRef]
39. Morales-Sánchez, D.; Tinoco-Valencia, R.; Kyndt, J.; Martinez, A. Heterotrophic growth of *Neochloris oleoabundans* using glucose as a carbon source. *Biotechnol. Biofuels* **2013**, *6*, 100. [CrossRef] [PubMed]
40. Leman, J. Oleaginous microorganisms: An assessment of the potential. In *Advances in Applied Microbiology*; Neidleman, S., Laskin, A., Eds.; Elsevier Academic Press: Cambridge, MA, USA, 1997; Volume 43, pp. 195–243.
41. Garcia-Ferris, C.; Rios, A.; Ascaso, C.; Moreno, J. Correlated biochemical and ultrastructural changes in nitrogen-starved *Euglena gracilis*. *J. Phycol.* **1996**, *32*, 953–963. [CrossRef]
42. Lillo, C.; Lea, U.; Ruoff, P. Nutrient depletion as a key factor for manipulating gene expression and product formation in different branches of the flavonoid pathway. *Plant Cell Environ.* **2008**, *31*, 587–601. [CrossRef]
43. Quiñones-Galvez, J.; Hernández de la Torre, M.; Quirós Molina, Y.; Capdesuñer Ruiz, Y.; Trujillo Sánchez, R. Factors controlling phenol content on *Theobroma cacao* callus culture. *Cultiv. Trop.* **2016**, *37*, 118–126.
44. Shetty, V.; Sibi, G. Relationship Between Total Phenolics Content and Antioxidant Activities of Microalgae Under Autotrophic, Heterotrophic and Mixotrophic Growth. *J. Food Resourc. Sci.* **2015**, *4*, 1–9.
45. Pulz, O.; Gross, W. Valuable products from biotechnology of microalgae. *Appl. Microbiol. Biotechnol.* **2004**, *65*, 635–648. [CrossRef]
46. Lippemeier, S.; Klaus, R.H.; Vanselow, K.H.; Hartig, P.; Colijn, F. In-line recording of PAM fluorescence of phytoplankton cultures as a new tool for studying effects of fluctuating nutrient supply on photosynthesis. *Eur. J. Phycol.* **2001**, *36*, 89–100. [CrossRef]
47. Apel, K.; Hirt, H. Reactive Oxygen Species: Metabolism, Oxidative Stress, and Signal Transduction. *Annu. Rev. Plant Biol.* **2004**, *55*, 373–399. [CrossRef] [PubMed]
48. Goiris, K.; Van Colen, W.; Wilches, I.; León-Tamariz, F.; De Cooman, L.; Muylaert, K. Impact of nutrient stress on antioxidant production in three species of microalgae. *Algal Res.* **2015**, *7*, 51–57. [CrossRef]
49. Alam, M.N.; Bristi, N.J.; Rafiquzzaman, M. Review on in vivo and in vitro methods evaluation of antioxidant activity. *Saudi Pharm. J.* **2013**, *21*, 143–152. [CrossRef] [PubMed]

50. Kumar, M.; Kumari, P.; Trivedi, N.; Shukla, M.K.; Gupta, V.; Reddy, C.R.K.; Jha, B. Minerals, PUFAs and antioxidant properties of some tropical seaweeds from Saurashtra coast of India. *J. App.l Phycol.* **2011**, *23*, 797–810. [CrossRef]
51. Surveswaran, S.; Cai, Y.Z.; Corke, H.; Sun, M. Systematic evaluation of natural phenolic antioxidants from 133 Indian medicinal plants. *Food Chem.* **2007**, *102*, 938–953. [CrossRef]
52. Jiménez-Escrig, A.; Jiménez-Jiménez, I.; Pulido, R.; Saura-Calixto, F. Antioxidant activity of fresh and processed edible seaweeds. *J. Sci. Food Agric.* **2001**, *81*, 530–534. [CrossRef]
53. Kováčik, J.; Klejdus, B.; Bačkor, M. Physiological Responses of *Scenedesmus quadricauda* (Chlorophyceae) to UV-A and UV-C Light. *Photochem. Photobiol.* **2010**, *86*, 612–616. [CrossRef]
54. Young, A.J. Factors that affect the carotenoid composition of higher plants and algae. In *Carotenoids in Photosynthesis*, 1st ed.; Young, A.J., Britton, G., Eds.; Springer: Dordrecht, The Netherlands, 1993; pp. 160–205.
55. Lapointe, B.E.; Duke, C.S. Biochemical strategies for growth of *Gracilaria tikvahiae* (Rhodophyta) in relation to light intensity and nitrogen availability. *J. Phycol.* **1984**, *20*, 488–495. [CrossRef]
56. Dogra, B.; Amna, S.; Il Park, Y.; Park, J.K. Biochemical Properties of Water Soluble Polysaccharides from Photosynthetic Marine Microalgae *Tetraselmis* Species. *Macromol. Res.* **2017**, *25*, 172–179. [CrossRef]
57. Kashif, S.A.; Hwang, Y.J.; Park, J.K. Potent biomedical applications of isolated polysaccharides from marine microalgae *Tetraselmis* species. *Bioproc. Biosyst. Eng.* **2018**, *41*, 1611–1620. [CrossRef]
58. Kirst, C.O. Salinity tolerance of eukaryotic marine algae. *Annu. Rev. Plant Physiol. Plant Mol. Biol.* **1989**, *40*, 21–53. [CrossRef]
59. Díaz Bayona, K.C.; Garcés, L. Effect of different media on exopolysaccharide and biomass production by the green microalga *Botryococcus braunii*. *J. Appl. Phycol.* **2014**, *26*, 2087–2095. [CrossRef]
60. Sun, L.; Wang, C.; Shi, Q.; Ma, C. Preparation of different molecular weight polysaccharides from *Porphyridium cruentum* and their antioxidant activities. *Int. J. Biol. Macromol.* **2009**, *45*, 42–47. [CrossRef]
61. Abdala, R.; Chabrillón, M.; Cabello-Pasini, A.; Gómez-Pinchetti, J.; Figueroa, F. Characterization of polysaccharides from *Hypnea spinella* (Gigartinales) and *Halopithys incurva* (Ceramiales) and their effect on RAW 264.7 macrophage activity. *J. Appl. Phycol.* **2011**, *23*, 523–528.
62. Fernando, I.P.S.; Sanjeewa, K.K.A.; Samarakoon, K.W.; Lee, W.W.; Kim, H.S.; Kim, E.A.; Gunasekara, U.K.D.S.S.; Abeytunga, D.T.U.; Nanayakkara, C.; de Silva, E.D.; et al. FTIR characterization and antioxidant activity of water soluble crude polysaccharides of Sri Lankan marine algae. *Algae 2017*, *2017*, 75–86. [CrossRef]
63. Parages, M.; Rico, R.; Abdala, R.; Chabrillón, M.; Sotiroudis, T.; Jiménez, C. Acidic polysaccharides of *Arthrospira* (Spirulina) *platensis* induce the synthesis of TNF-α in RAW macrophages. *J. Appl. Phycol.* **2012**, *24*, 1537–1546. [CrossRef]
64. Cabassi, F.; Casu, B.; Perlin, A.S. Infrared absorption and raman scattering of sulfate groups of heparin and related glycosaminoglycans in aqueous solution. *Carbohydr. Res.* **1978**, *63*, 1–11. [CrossRef]
65. Pereira, L.; Amado, A.M.; Critchley, A.T.; van de Velde, F.; Ribeiro-Claro, P.J.A. Identification of selected seaweed polysaccharides (phycocolloids) by vibrational spectroscopy (FTIR-ATR and FT-Raman). *Food Hydrocoll.* **2009**, *23*, 1903–1909. [CrossRef]
66. Pereira, L.; Gheda, S.F.; Ribeiro-Claro, P.J.A. Analysis by Vibrational Spectroscopy of Seaweed Polysaccharides with Potential Use in Food, Pharmaceutical, and Cosmetic Industries. *Int. J. Carbohydr. Chem.* **2013**, *2013*, 1–7. [CrossRef]
67. Pereira, L.; Sousa, A.; Coelho, H.; Amado, A.M.; Ribeiro-Claro, P.J.A. Use of FTIR, FT-Raman and 13 C-NMR spectroscopy for identification of some seaweed phycocolloids. *Biomol. Eng.* **2003**, *20*, 223–228. [CrossRef]
68. Meng, Y.; Yao, C.; Xue, S.; Yang, H. Application of fourier transform infrared (FT-IR) spectroscopy in determination of microalgal compositions. *Bioresour. Technol.* **2014**, *151*, 347–354. [CrossRef]
69. Kermanshahi-Pour, A.; Sommer, T.J.; Anastas, P.T.; Zimmerman, J.B. Enzymatic and acid hydrolysis of *Tetraselmis suecica* for polysaccharide characterization. *Bioresour. Technol.* **2014**, *173*, 415–421. [CrossRef] [PubMed]
70. Becker, B.; Hard, K.; Melkonian, M.; Kamerling, J.P.G.; Vliegenthart, J.F. Identification of 3-deoxy-manno-2-octulosonic acid, 3-deoxy-5-O-methyl-rnanno-2-octulosonic acid and 3-deoxy-lyxo-2-heptulosaric acid in the cell wall (theca) of the green alga *Tetraselmis striata* Butcher (Prasinophyceae). *Eur. J. Biochem.* **1989**, *182*, 153–160. [CrossRef] [PubMed]
71. Becker, B.; Lommerse, J.P.M.; Melkonian, M.; Kamerling, J.P.; Vliegenthart, J.F.G. The structure of an acidic trisaccharide component from a cell wall polysaccharide preparation of the green alga *Tetraselmis striata* Butcher. *Carbohydr. Res.* **1995**, *267*, 313–321. [CrossRef]

72. Becker, B.; Melkonian, M.; Kamerling, J.P. The cell wall (theca) of *Tetraselmis striata* (Chlorophyta): Macromolecular compositionand structural elementsof the complex polysaccharides. *J. Phycol.* **1998**, *34*, 779–787. [CrossRef]
73. Xiao, R.; Zheng, Y. Overview of microalgal extracellular polymeric substances (EPS) and their applications. *Biotechnol. Adv.* **2016**, *34*, 1225–1244. [CrossRef]
74. Chen, X.; Song, L.; Wang, H.; Liu, S.; Yu, H.; Wang, X.; Li, R.; Liu, T.; Li, P. Partial Characterization, the Immune Modulation and Anticancer Activities of Sulfated Polysaccharides from Filamentous Microalgae *Tribonema* sp. *Molecules* **2019**, *24*, 322. [CrossRef]
75. Yang, S.; Wan, H.; Wang, R.; Hao, D. Sulfated polysaccharides from *Phaeodactylum tricornutum*: Isolation, structural characteristics, and inhibiting HepG2 growth activity in vitro. *PeerJ.* **2019**, *7*, e6409. [CrossRef]
76. Abd El Baky, H.; Hanna El Baz, K.; El-Latife, S. Induction of Sulfated Polysaccharides in *Spirulina platensis* as Response to Nitrogen Concentration and its Biological Evaluation. *J. Aquac. Res. Dev.* **2013**, *5*, 1–8.
77. Sun, L.; Wang, L.; Zhou, Y. Immunomodulation and antitumor activities of different-molecular-weight polysaccharides from *Porphyridium cruentum*. *Carbohydr. Polym.* **2012**, *87*, 1206–1210. [CrossRef]
78. Gardeva, E.; Toshkova, R.; Yossifova, L.; Minkova, K.; Gigova, L. Cytotoxic and apoptogenic potential of red microalgal polysaccharides. *Biotechnol. Biotechnol. Equip.* **2012**, *26*, 3167–3172. [CrossRef]
79. Yao, W.Z.; Veeraperumal, S.; Qiu, H.M.; Chen, X.Q.; Cheong, K.L. Anti-cancer effects of *Porphyra haitanensis* polysaccharides on human colon cancer cells via cell cycle arrest and apoptosis without causing adverse effects in vitro. *3 Biotech.* **2020**, *10*, 386. [CrossRef] [PubMed]
80. Nani, B.D.; Franchin, M.; Lazarini, J.G.; Freires, I.A.; da Cunha, M.G.; Bueno-Silva, B.; de Alencar, S.M.; Murata, R.M.; Rosalen, P.L. Isoflavonoids from Brazilian red propolis down-regulate the expression of cancer-related target proteins: A pharmacogenomic analysis. *Phytother. Res.* **2018**, *32*, 750–754. [CrossRef] [PubMed]
81. Guillard, R. Culture of phytoplankton for feeding marine invertebrate animals. In *Culture of Marine Invertebrates*, 1st ed.; Smith, W., Chanley, M., Eds.; Springer: Boston, MA, USA, 1975; pp. 29–60.
82. Sun, Y.; Wang, H.; Guo, G.; Pu, Y.; Yan, B. The isolation and antioxidant activity of polysaccharides from the marine microalgae *Isochrysis galbana*. *Carbohydr. Polym.* **2014**, *113*, 22–31. [CrossRef] [PubMed]
83. Morris Quevedo, H.J.; Martínez Manrique, C.E.; Abdala Díaz, R.T.; Cobas Pupo, G. Evidencias preliminares de la actividad inmunomoduladora de la fracción polisacárida de origen marino Pc-1. *Rev. Cuba. Oncol.* **2000**, *16*, 171–177.
84. Arredondo-Vega, B.O.; Voltolina, D. Concentración, recuento celular y tasa de crecimiento. In *Métodos y Herramientas Analíticas en la Evaluación de la Biomasa Microalgal*, 1st ed.; Arredondo, B.O., Voltolina, D., Eds.; CIBNOR: La Paz, B.C.S., Mexico, 2007; pp. 21–29.
85. Lourenço, S.O.; Barbarino, E.; Lavín, P.L.; Lanfer Marquez, U.M.; Aidar, E. Distribution of intracellular nitrogen in marine microalgae: Calculation of new nitrogen-to-protein conversion factors. *Eur. J. Phycol.* **2004**, *39*, 17–32. [CrossRef]
86. Folch, J.; Less, M.; Sloane Stanley, G.H. A Simple method for the isolation and purification of total lipides from animal tissues. *J. Biol. Chem.* **1957**, *226*, 497–509. [PubMed]
87. Dubois, M.; Gilles, K.A.; Hamilton, J.K.; Rebers, P.A.; Smith, F. Colorimetric method for determination of sugars and related substances. *Anal. Biochem.* **1956**, *28*, 350–356. [CrossRef]
88. Folin, O.; Ciocalteau, V. On tyrosine and tryptophane determinations in proteins. *J. Biol. Chem.* **1927**, *73*, 627–648.
89. Ritchie, R.J. Consistent sets of spectrophotometric chlorophyll equations for acetone, methanol and ethanol solvents. *Photosynth. Res.* **2006**, *89*, 27–41. [CrossRef] [PubMed]
90. Ritchie, R.J. Universal chlorophyll equations for estimating chlorophylls a, b, c, and d and total chlorophylls in natural assemblages of photosynthetic organisms using acetone, methanol, or ethanol solvents. *Photosynthetica* **2008**, *46*, 115–126. [CrossRef]
91. Strickland, J.D.H.; Parsons, T.R. *A Practical Handbook of Seawater Analysis*, 2nd ed.; Fisheries Research Board of Canada: Ottawa, ON, Canada, 2008; pp. 1–310.
92. Re, R.; Pellegrini, N.; Proteggente, A.; Pannala, A.; Yang, M.; Rice-Evans, C. Antioxidant activity applying an improved ABTS radical cation decolorization assay. *Free Radic. Bio. Med.* **1999**, *26*, 1231–1237. [CrossRef]
93. Vijayabaskar, P.; Vaseela, N. In vitro antioxidant properties of sulfated polysaccharide from brown marine algae *Sargassum tenerrimum*. *Asian Pac. J. Trop. Dis.* **2012**, S890–S896. [CrossRef]

94. Brand-Williams, W.; Cuvelier, M.E.; Berset, C. Use of a Free Radical Method to Evaluate Antioxidant Activity. *Lebensm. Wiss. Technol.* **1995**, *28*, 25–30. [CrossRef]
95. Underwood, A.J. *Experiments in Ecology: Their Logical Design and Interpretation Using Analysis of Variance*, 1st ed.; Cambridge University Press: Cambridge, UK, 1997; pp. 1–522.

Publisher's Note: MDPI stays neutral with regard to jurisdictional claims in published maps and institutional affiliations.

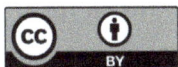
© 2020 by the authors. Licensee MDPI, Basel, Switzerland. This article is an open access article distributed under the terms and conditions of the Creative Commons Attribution (CC BY) license (http://creativecommons.org/licenses/by/4.0/).

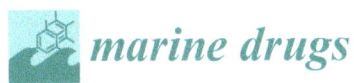

Article

One Step Forward towards the Development of Eco-Friendly Antifouling Coatings: Immobilization of a Sulfated Marine-Inspired Compound

Cátia Vilas-Boas [1,2], Francisca Carvalhal [1,2], Beatriz Pereira [3], Sílvia Carvalho [4], Emília Sousa [1,2], Madalena M. M. Pinto [1,2], Maria José Calhorda [3], Vitor Vasconcelos [2,5], Joana R. Almeida [2], Elisabete R. Silva [3,*] and Marta Correia-da-Silva [1,2,*]

1. Laboratório de Química Orgânica e Farmacêutica, Departamento de Ciências Químicas, Faculdade de Farmácia, Universidade do Porto, R. Jorge de Viterbo Ferreira 228, 4050-313 Porto, Portugal; catiaboas94@gmail.com (C.V.-B.); francisca.carvalhal@gmail.com (F.C.); esousa@ff.up.pt (E.S.); madalena@ff.up.pt (M.M.M.P.)
2. CIIMAR—Centro Interdisciplinar de Investigação Marinha e Ambiental, Avenida General Norton de Matos, S/N, 4450-208 Matosinhos, Portugal; vmvascon@fc.up.pt (V.V.); joana.reis.almeida@gmail.com (J.R.A.)
3. BioISI—Instituto de Biosistemas e Ciências Integrativas, Departamento de Química e Bioquímica, Faculdade de Ciências, Universidade de Lisboa, Campo Grande, Lisboa, 1749-016 Portugal; beatrizmmgpereira@gmail.com (B.P.); mjcalhorda@fc.ul.pt (M.J.C.)
4. CQB—Centro de Química e Bioquímica, Departamento de Química e Bioquímica, Faculdade de Ciências, Universidade de Lisboa, Campo Grande, Lisboa, 1749-016 Lisboa, Portugal; scfcarvalho@fc.ul.pt
5. Departamento de Biologia, Faculdade de Ciências, Universidade do Porto, Rua do Campo Alegre S/N, 4169-007 Porto, Portugal
* Correspondence: ersilva@fc.ul.pt (E.R.S.); m_correiadasilva@ff.up.pt (M.C.-d.-S.)

Received: 18 August 2020; Accepted: 23 September 2020; Published: 25 September 2020

Abstract: Marine biofouling represents a global economic and ecological challenge and few eco-friendly antifouling agents are available. The aim of this work was to establish the proof of concept that a recently synthesized nature-inspired compound (gallic acid persulfate, GAP) can act as an eco-friendly and effective antifoulant when immobilized in coatings through a non-release strategy, promoting a long-lasting antifouling effect. The synthesis of GAP was optimized to provide quantitative yields. GAP water solubility was assessed, showing values higher than 1000 mg/mL. GAP was found to be stable in sterilized natural seawater with a half-life (DT_{50}) of 7 months. GAP was immobilized into several commercial coatings, exhibiting high compatibility with different polymeric matrices. Leaching assays of polydimethylsiloxane and polyurethane-based marine coatings containing GAP confirmed that the chemical immobilization of GAP was successful, since releases up to fivefold lower than the conventional releasing systems of polyurethane-based marine coatings were observed. Furthermore, coatings containing immobilized GAP exhibited the most auspicious anti-settlement effect against *Mytilus galloprovincialis* larvae for the maximum exposure period (40 h) in laboratory trials. Overall, GAP promises to be an agent capable of improving the antifouling activity of several commercial marine coatings with desirable environmental properties.

Keywords: biofouling; marine coatings; anti-settlement; chemical synthesis; sulfated; gallic acid; eco-friendly

1. Introduction

Marine biofouling consists of the settlement and gradual accumulation of micro- and macro-organisms, such as bacteria, fungi, spores of algae, and invertebrate larvae in water submerged surfaces [1–3]. However, despite this natural process starting with the attachment and proliferation of bacteria, it is the growth of macrofouling organisms that most concerns marine industries. Their dense layers can cause a reduction in or even blockage of water flow in pipes, mechanical damage, corrosion, and the failure of equipment [4]. In other words, marine biofouling can increase maintenance costs and fuel consumption [5,6].

Chemical control is the principal strategy to combat this issue, combining traditional antifouling (AF) coatings, as is the case of polydimethylsiloxane (PDMS) and polyurethane (PU)-based coatings, with biocides, which are released over time [7,8]. Although most of them are presented as non-persistent biocides, several occurrence studies have concluded that, in fact, booster biocides persist, owing to their high release in biocide-release-based AF coatings [9–12]. In addition, due to their low water solubility and hydrophobic behavior, booster biocides tend to bioaccumulate, causing environmental damage [13–15]. Fortunately, there is increasing concern about the influence of copper and booster biocides in the marine environment and the effort to find ecological alternatives has led many researchers to develop greener AF approaches in order to reduce biocide release and consequently their persistence in the ecosystem [16–20]. A good AF agent must prevent fouling without persisting at concentrations greater than those that can cause detrimental effects to the environment.

A large variety of microorganisms and sessile marine organisms, such as sponges, corals, and algae, usually free of fouling on their surfaces, has been described to produce secondary metabolites to fight this natural process [21], as is the case of zosteric acid (ZA), a sulfated phenolic acid produced by the seagrass *Zostera marina* [22,23]. Inspired by the ZA structure, AF properties of a small library of synthetic sulfated small molecules were studied and gallic acid persulfate (GAP) was found to be one of the most promising compounds [24]. Furthermore, gallic acid, its starting material, is commercially available and easily accessible since it can be obtained from several sources, such as winery waste [25]. In contrast to ZA, GAP showed anti-settlement activity against the adhesive larvae of *Mytilus galloprovincialis*, one of the most aggressive invasive species in the world, according to the International Union for Conservation of Nature (IUCN) [26], without causing ecotoxicity against this species and other non-target species (Figure 1) [24].

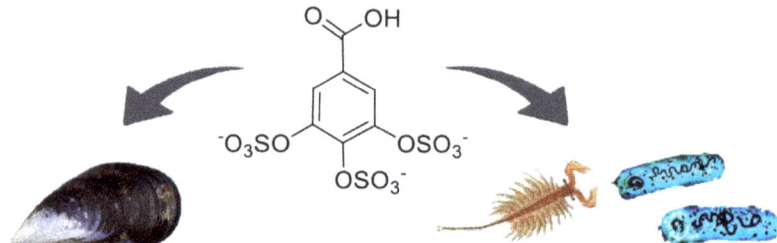

Figure 1. Antifouling (AF) activity and ecotoxicity previously discovered for gallic acid persulfate (GAP) [24].

To assess GAP suitability as an AF agent, it is necessary to evaluate compound stability and degradation pathways, optimize its large-scale synthesis, and analyze its behavior after incorporation in selected coating formulations. In this study, both the solubility of GAP in ultra-pure water (UPW) and in sterilized natural seawater (snSW), as well as the stability of sulfate groups after exposure to varying conditions of light and temperature for a period of several months, were examined. GAP synthesis was optimized through a microwave (MW) reaction to obtain high amounts of the compound and allow further immobilization in traditional marine coatings. Coating formulations with new synthesized GAP were developed using both direct incorporation (DI) and chemical immobilization (CI) strategies into two representative marine coatings: PDMS and PU-based coatings. The purpose of the chemical immobilization of GAP was to achieve maximal compatibility between this polar molecule and polymeric coatings, as well as provide long-lasting antifouling effects with a non-release strategy. Leaching assays were performed to confirm the minimal release of GAP into the aquatic environment.

As the targets of any preventive technology are the colonizing stages [27], the settlement inhibition of *Mytilus galloprovincialis* larvae on the several GAP-based coating formulations was evaluated.

During these studies, two analytical methods were developed in order to: (1) directly analyze this sulfated polar compound in snSW, through an ion pair reversed-phase high performance liquid chromatography (IP-RP-HPLC) method (stability assays) [28] and (2) concentrate and extract this analyte from the leached artificial seawater (ASW), through a weak anionic exchange (WAX) method preceding IP-RP-HPLC quantification (leaching assays).

2. Results and Discussion

2.1. Solubility in Water

The solubility of GAP was higher than 1000 mg/mL at 24 ± 1 in UPW and snSW, being classified according to the USP Pharmacopeia as a "very soluble" compound [29]. The high water solubility of GAP is in accordance with the reduced value (−7.02) of its *n*-octanol/water partition coefficient ($logK_{ow}$) previously calculated with EPISUITE [24]. This suggests that water will retain the compound in solution, reinforcing the low affinity of GAP for sediments and fatty tissues, which makes GAP an eco-friendly candidate to be incorporated in coatings [22,24].

2.2. Optimization of the IP-RP-HPLC Method

An IP-RP-HPLC method was developed to quantify GAP in UPW and snSW. First, several mobile phases containing different proportions of acetonitrile and acidified water (0.1% acetic acid) were investigated. However, the retention factor (k) was not satisfactory (less than 1), with GAP overlapping with the solvent front. As the retention of this charged molecule was not achieved by regular reversed-phase, a mobile phase containing an aqueous solution of 25 mM of tetrabutylammonium bromide (TBA-Br) and acetonitrile (38:62 *v/v*) was used to favor ion pairing, and consequently suitable k values between 1-10 could be reached [28]. The ion pairing of GAP dissolved in UPW was accomplished, with an acceptable k value of 1. However, in snSW a k of 0 was still observed, even using different proportions of the mobile phase. In order to assure retention (k ≠ 0), using the same aqueous mobile phase containing TBA-Br and acetonitrile (38:62 *v/v*), a pre-treatment of the sample was carried out before injection, diluting GAP dissolved in snSW with 60 mM of TBA-Br in a proportion of 1:3, leading to ion pairing with a desirable k value of one.

2.3. Stability of Sulfate Groups in Water

To assess the stability of GAP in water, its half-life (DT_{50}) was evaluated in UPW and snSW. GAP was exposed to several stress conditions (4 °C, 18 °C and r.t. (24 ± 1) in the absence and presence of natural light) in order to mimic different natural environmental conditions and its stability was determined at 0, 2 and 9 months.

In UPW, the concentration of GAP significantly decreases after the first 2 months (except at 4 °C in darkness), but it remains approximately constant during the following consecutive months, for a total of 9 months (Figure 2), suggesting the chemical stability of the sulfate linkage (without significant differences ($p < 0.05$) between the initial time and the ninth month).

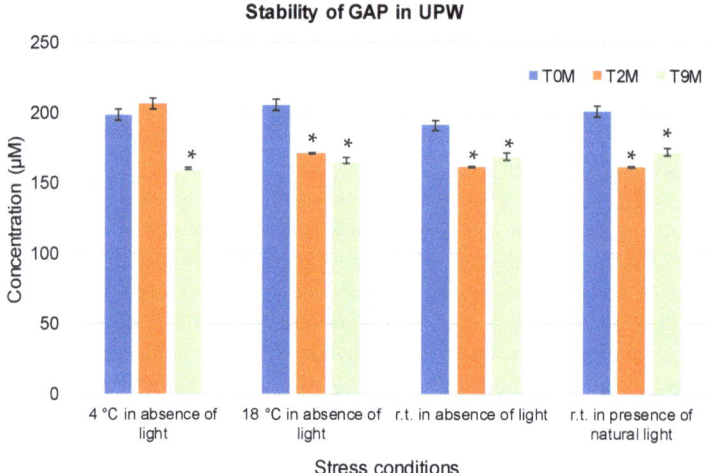

Figure 2. Stability of gallic acid persulfate (GAP) dissolved in ultra-pure water (UPW) (200 µM) and exposed to several stress conditions over a period of 9 months. * Indicates significant differences at $p < 0.05$ (Dunnett test) against the negative control (initial time (T0M), blue bar). T0M: initial time; T2M: two months; T9M: nine months).

After 9 months in snSW, GAP was abiotically degraded, reaching a significant 50% degradation ($p < 0.05$) from which a half-life (DT_{50}) value of 7 months in all tested stress conditions was calculated (Figure 3). This study also suggests that photolysis may not accelerate GAP degradation, since the degradation rate did not increase in the presence of light and there are non-significant differences ($p < 0.05$). In the future, the identification of transformation products by liquid chromatography associated to high resolution Mass Spectrometry (LC-MS), as well as their ecotoxicological evaluation, will be performed, providing information to regulatory authorities.

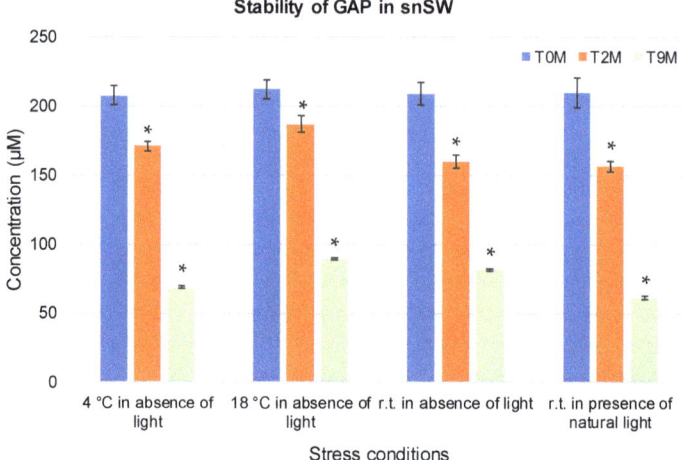

Figure 3. Stability of gallic acid persulfate (GAP) dissolved in sterilized natural seawater (snSW) (200 µM), exposed to the several stress conditions over a period of 9 months. * Indicates significant differences at $p < 0.05$ (Dunnett test) against the negative control (T0M, blue bar). T0M: initial time; T2M: two months; T9M: nine months).

2.4. GAP-Based Marine Coatings

2.4.1. Synthesis Optimization

The synthesis of GAP was optimized to obtain sufficient amounts of this product in order to prepare marine coating formulations. A reproducible and feasible one-step synthesis of GAP was accomplished by sulfation of gallic acid with the triethylamine sulfur trioxide adduct (TEA·SO$_3$) and triethylamine (TEA), in dimethylformamide (DMF), under MW heating (Scheme 1). Gallic acid is a commercially available and affordable raw material and it can be obtained from several sources, such as winery waste [25].

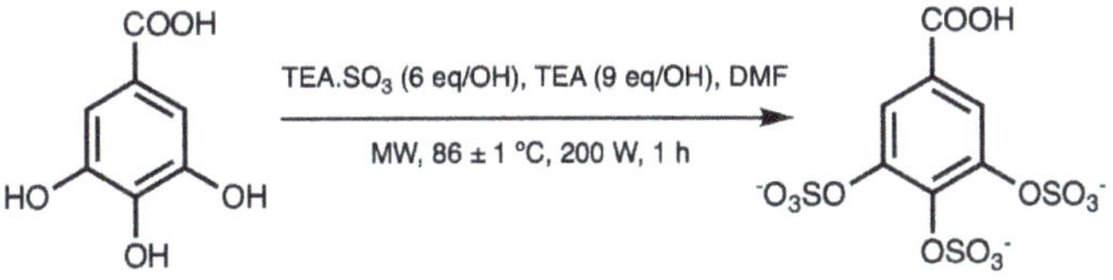

Scheme 1. Synthesis of gallic acid persulfate (GAP).

MW irradiation is a potent green chemistry tool and, in the last decade, also emerged as a new alternative approach to obtain sulfated derivatives [30–33]. The technique offers a simple, clean, fast, efficient, and economic strategy for the synthesis of a large number of organic molecules [34]. MW heating increased the efficiency of the synthetic method, demanding lower reaction times when compared to conventional heating, and significantly increased the yield of the reaction (Table 1).

Table 1. Comparative conditions for sulfation of gallic acid.

Reaction	Reagents	Solvent	Reaction Conditions	Reaction Time	Yields
Previous synthesis [35]	TEA·SO$_3$ (2 eq/OH)	DMA	Conventional heating 65 °C	24 h	36%
Optimized synthesis	TEA·SO$_3$ (6 eq/OH) TEA (9 eq/OH)	DMF	MW 200 W 86 °C	1 h	98%

TEA·SO$_3$: triethylamine-sulfur trioxide adduct; TEA: triethylamine; DMA: dimethylacetamide; DMF: dimethylformamide; h: hours; MW: microwave.

Additionally, the use of a free base in the reaction mixture allowed us to overcome the difficult persulfation of gallic acid, a tri-hydroxylated molecule. After the reaction, more triethylamine (33 eq/OH) was added to ensure the conversion of the sulfate groups into triethylamine salts, which were more easily separated in oil form in the crude product and led to an improved yield when compared to the previous purification process. The instability of the triethylamine salts was then overcome by quick conversion into sodium salts with sodium acetate. The grade of the newly synthesized GAP was similar to the grade of previous GAP (HPLC, Figure S1). The infrared and ^{1}H nuclear magnetic resonance (NMR) spectra were in accordance with the literature [35].

2.4.2. GAP Immobilization Strategies

To evaluate the potential of GAP as an AF agent in real coating systems, this compound was, for the first time, directly incorporated (DI) and chemically immobilized (CI) into two representative marine coatings: PDMS and PU-based coatings. The direct incorporation allows us to assess the feasibility of the new synthetized GAP as an AF agent in conventional release AF coating systems, while the chemical immobilization strategy demonstrates the potential of GAP to be grafted in polymeric non-release coating systems [36], thus promoting long-lasting effects in the generated protective coating compared with the short lifetime of the conventional releasing systems.

The CI GAP was promoted by the addition and blending of the trimethylolpropane triaziridine propionate crosslinker (TZA) in the coating formulations. TZA is a versatile crosslinker which reacts with functional groups of coating components carrying an active hydrogen (e.g., alkoxy), as happens with the carboxyl function in the GAP structure. The immobilization effectiveness was confirmed by analyzing the interaction of TZA with the GAP AF agent through Fourier Transform Infrared Spectroscopy (FTIR) analysis. Figure 4 shows the obtained GAP derivative (GAP–TZA) and the spectra of GAP and TZA for comparison purposes. The assignment of the spectra was carried out by calculating the vibrational spectra of GAP and TZA and comparing them to the spectra of GAP, TZA, and the GAP–TZA derivative (DFT, ADF/BP86/TZ2P; see structures and computational details in Figure S2 in Supplementary Materials).

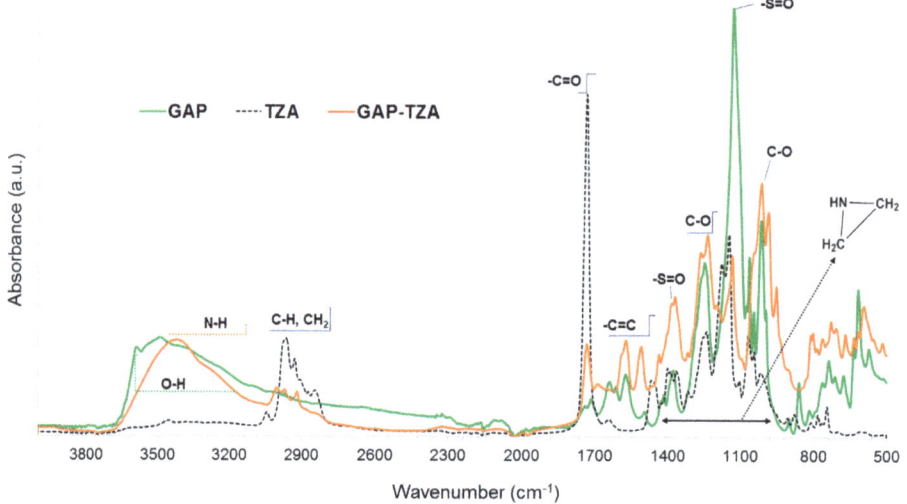

Figure 4. Normalized infrared spectra (FTIR-ATR) of gallic acid persulfate (GAP, green line), triaziridine propionate crosslinker (TZA, black line) and GAP–TZA derivative (brown line).

The FTIR spectrum of GAP clearly shows the broadened characteristic band assigned to the hydroxyl stretching vibration frequencies of the carboxylic acid group, ranging from 3600 cm^{-1} to 3200 cm^{-1}, with a maximum at 3494 cm^{-1}. It also shows vibrational modes between 1750 cm^{-1} and 1700 cm^{-1}, assigned to carbonyl stretching (C=O) of the carboxylic acid function, at 1612 cm^{-1} and 1571 cm^{-1}, assigned to the aromatic C=C stretching vibrations, and from 1415 cm^{-1} to 1380 cm^{-1}, assigned to S=O stretching. The bands from 1338 cm^{-1} to 1200 cm^{-1} correspond to the characteristic acyl (–C–O) stretching vibrations and can overlap with the asymmetrical stretching vibrations of the aryl sulfate. Lower frequency vibrational modes, ranging from 1010–1100 cm^{-1}, are attributed to the C–O stretching vibration, and the strong band at 1134 cm^{-1} to the symmetrical stretching of aryl sulfate (S=O). Bands between 550–590 cm^{-1} and 617–650 cm^{-1} can be assigned to SO_3 bending vibrations, and in the 757–838 cm^{-1} range to S–(OC) stretching vibrations.

The TZA spectrum shows an intense band at 1751 cm^{-1} assigned to the C=O stretching vibrational modes, corresponding to the carbonyl group of saturated aliphatic esters, and bands ranging from 1400 to 1040 cm^{-1} assigned to the stretching vibrations of aziridine rings.

The spectrum of the GAP–TZA derivative additionally shows a distinct band at 3400 – 3300 cm^{-1}, characteristic of the amine stretching vibrations, suggesting that the opening of the aziridine ring of TZA took place upon reaction with GAP. Moreover, the shift in the carbonyl stretching vibrations (from 1736 cm^{-1} in TZA and 1754 cm^{-1} in GAP) to 1732 cm^{-1} in GAP–TZA suggests the intermolecular bonding of TZA to carboxyl groups of GAP to yield amino-ester bonds (Scheme 2) [37].

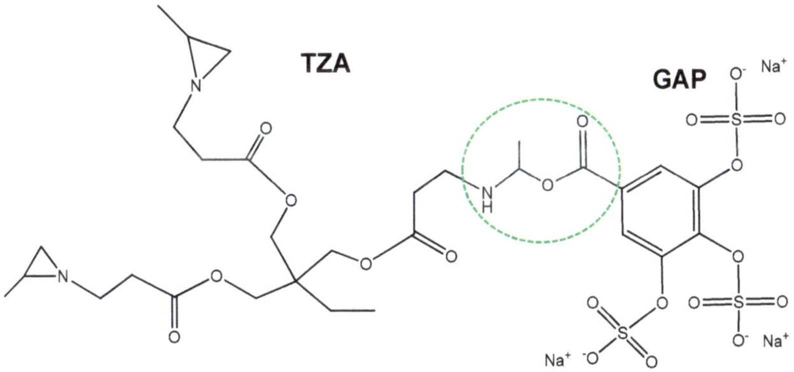

Scheme 2. Illustration of a GAP–TZA derivative linkage obtained upon direct reaction of gallic acid persulfate (GAP) with triaziridine propionate crosslinker (TZA).

^{1}H and ^{13}C nuclear magnetic resonance (NMR) spectra of GAP, TZA, and the GAP–TZA derivative were also obtained in DMSO-d_6 (c.f. SI). Despite the poor solubility of GAP–TZA and the low resolution of the spectrum, the identification of some signals reinforces the FTIR results. The chemical shifts at $\delta \cong 7.50$ ppm correspond to the aromatic protons of the GAP while the chemical shifts from 0.80–4.80 ppm indicate the presence of a TZA moiety, according to the ^{1}H NMR of a similar compound, TMPTA-AZ [37]. In the GAP–TZA ^{1}H NMR spectrum, the signal corresponding to the aromatic protons of the gallic moiety was observed at 7.52 ppm, which was more protected than in free GAP (7.85 ppm), as expected. An additional resonance observed in this region (7.37 ppm) could be attributed to a minor impurity (from reagents). Its significance may be enhanced due to the low solubility of GAP–TZA. The new signal at 1.63 ppm (^{1}H NMR) and 25.91 ppm (^{13}C) assigned to C14 (Figure S6, SM), as well as a low intensity signal at 2.01 ppm (NH) in the ^{1}H NMR, suggest that the reaction between GAP and TZA occurred with the opening of the ring. Additionally, the ^{1}H and ^{13}C NMR spectra also indicate that the reaction did not occur in all three aziridine units, since it is still possible to observe signals corresponding to those units (Figures S1–S4): 1.31–1.39 ppm (H_5), 34.25 ppm (C_5); 1.01 ppm (H_4), 18.70 ppm (C_4); 1.17 and 1.29 ppm (H_6 and $H_{6'}$), 34.21 ppm (C_6).

2.4.3. Marine Coating Formulations

The main goal was to achieve compatible behavior between the GAP compound and the selected coating systems (DI and CI), to determine the limiting GAP content supported by each system. Several formulations of the coatings were optimized in an iterative process considering different GAP contents, solvent compatibilities, and incorporation of additional paint additives. Finally, the optimum GAP concentration was selected as the one that did not damage the main paint properties, i.e., the formulation looked the same as the control (coating system without the immobilization of GAP), Figure S7. The most promising optimized formulations are presented in Table 2 and were selected to pursue further evaluations.

Table 2. Marine coating formulations with gallic acid persulfate (GAP).

Coating Formulation	Polymeric Matrix	Base/Curing Agent Ratio (v/v)	GAP Content (wt.%)	TZA Content (wt.%)
GAP-DI/PU	Polyurethane	2/1	1.99 ± 0.02	—
GAP-CI/PU	Polyurethane	2/1	2.05 ± 0.02	2.06 ± 0.02
GAP-DI/PDMS	Polydimethylsiloxane	17.8/2.2	0.55 ± 0.02	—
GAP-CI/PDMS	Polydimethylsiloxane	17.8/2.2	0.56 ± 0.02	2.05 ± 0.02

CI: chemically immobilized; DI: directly incorporated; PDMS: polydimethylsiloxane; PU: Polyurethane; TZA: triaziridine propionate crosslinker.

2.4.4. GAP Quantification in Leaching Water Samples

To evaluate the effectiveness of the CI strategy in minimizing the release of GAP from the coatings into the aquatic environment, leaching tests were performed using polyvinylchloride (PVC) plates coated with the selected marine coatings formulations. After a period of 45 days, the released GAP was extracted from leaching water samples through an optimized weak anionic exchange (WAX) methodology and then dissolved in UPW. The WAX stationary phase possesses weak groups (secondary amines), which are activated at a reduced working pH, creating a reversible interaction with strongly acidic, acidic and neutral compounds, allowing their concentration and extraction. Therefore, a low pH loading step (pH < 5) will ionize the stationary phase to facilitate the retention of GAP in the leaching water, while the remaining impurities are discarded. The elution of GAP is achieved by increasing the pH to >11, neutralizing the stationary phase. Table 3 shows the amount of detected GAP after quantification by the previously established IP-RP-HPLC method.

Table 3. Gallic acid persulfate (GAP) amount released from marine coatings prepared by direct incorporation (DI) and chemical immobilization (CI) strategies into artificial seawater (ASW), after an immersion period of 45 days.

Polymeric Coatings(n)	Immobilization	GAP Amount in Coated PVC Plates (mg) *	Amount of Detected GAP Leached to Waters after 45 Days (mg) *	Content of Released GAP from Coated PVC Plates (wt.%) *
GAP-DI/PU(2)	Direct	26.90 ± 2.60	4.95 ± 0.25	18.49 ± 0.86
GAP-CI/PU(2)	Chemical	34.00 ± 1.7	1.37 ± 0.06	4.02 ± 0.03
GAP-DI/PDMS(2)	Direct	6.75 ± 0.25	1.39 ± 0.02	20.59 ± 1.00
GAP-CI/PDMS(2)	Chemical	4.95 ± 0.75	0.55 ± 0.13	10.94 ± 0.90

(n): number of replicates; PDMS: polydimethylsiloxane; PU: polyurethane; PVC: polyvinyl chloride. * mean values ± standard deviation of two independent experiences.

After a period of 45 days, the content of GAP present in the several leaching water samples, after DI in PU and PDMS coatings, was approximately 20% (Table 3). However, after CI, the percentage of GAP released from PDMS coating was only 11% (two times lower than DI in PDMS coatings), and from PU coatings 4% (almost five times lower than DI in PU coatings). These results demonstrate the high effectiveness of the chemical immobilization to retain this water-soluble compound in marine coatings, compared to the DI strategy. This phenomenon is also clearly more pronounced for a polyurethane-based matrix, which may be explained by the higher chemical compatibility of the GAP–TZA derivative functionality with a polyurethane system, associated with the intrinsic reactivity of aziridine and its possible cross-link promotion with the highly alkoxy-reactive polyurethane system, thus allowing us to reach higher agent content in the formulations (Table 3) [17].

2.4.5. Anti-Settlement Behavior of GAP after Incorporation in Coatings

In order to evaluate the ability of the different GAP-containing marine coatings to prevent the attachment of mussel larvae, the anti-settlement response was evaluated at lab scale in a bioassay using *Mytilus galloprovincialis* larvae (Figure 5).

PU marine coating containing CI GAP seems to be effective against the settlement of mussel larvae, inhibiting larval settlement after both 15 h (−50%) and 40 h (−80%), in wells with this coating, compared to the control (PU). Although the individual variability of the larvae responses does not allow significantly different results against the control, the obtained settlement inhibition rates still represent a good indicator of the GAP AF potential in marine coatings. In contrast, PU marine coating containing DI GAP did not behave differently from the control. Since this conventional insoluble PU-based coating matrix acts mainly through a leaching effect [38], this result may indicate that the leaching rate and/or available GAP concentration in test media and on the outer surface of the coating is not enough to provide an effective AF action. The antifouling mechanisms involved, for instance, following leaching and/or contact strategies, would require a deep reformulation of coatings and further characterization, which go beyond the scope of this work.

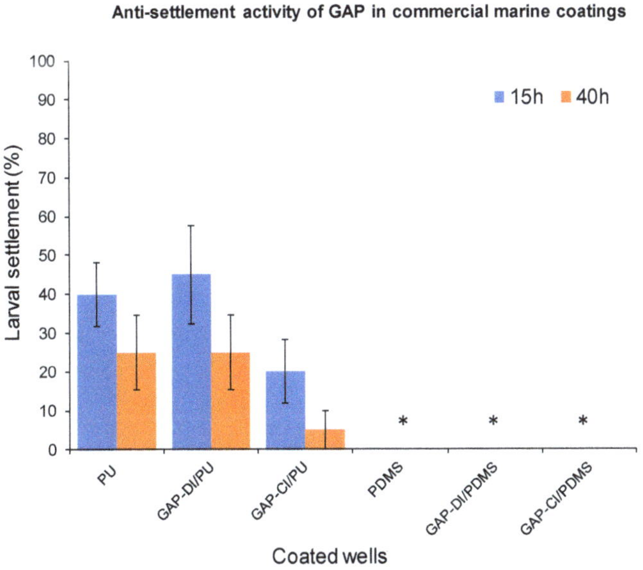

Anti-settlement activity of GAP in commercial marine coatings

Figure 5. Anti-settlement activity of gallic acid persulfate (GAP) towards *Mytilus galloprovincialis* larvae after direct incorporation (DI) and chemical immobilization (CI) in commercial marine coatings. PU: polyurethane; PDMS: polydimethylsiloxane; h: hours. * No larval settlement was observed for the PDMS-based coated wells.

In the experiments with the PDMS-based AF marine coating formulations, a high anti-settlement effect was observed in the wells coated with the control formulation, which can be explained by the coating's intrinsic non-stick properties [39]. This experimental approach with PDMS is thus not informative regarding the efficacy of GAP, but contributes to the understanding that this matrix is, per se, highly effective against mussel larvae attachment.

Thus, to better assess the influence of the presence of GAP in the coatings' anti-settlement properties, and also to overcome any masked effect from the intrinsic properties of the marine coatings, complementary assays with other optimized formulations of acrylic (AV) and room-temperature-vulcanizing (RTV)-PDMS-based non-marine coatings, were performed (c.f. Table 4). In the future, in situ tests will be performed to demonstrate the real potential applications of GAP-containing marine coatings in different AF systems worldwide.

Table 4. Non-marine coatings formulations with immobilized gallic acid persulfate (GAP).

Coating Formulation	Polymeric Matrix	Base/Curing Agent Ratio (v/v)	GAP Content (wt.%)	TZA Content (wt.%)
GAP-DI/AV	Acrylic	3/1	0.56 ± 0.02	—
GAP-CI/AV	Acrylic	3/1	0.56 ± 0.02	2.46 ± 0.03
GAP-DI/AV	Acrylic	3/1	1.00 ± 0.02	—
GAP-CI/AV	Acrylic	3/1	1.00 ± 0.02	2.42 ± 0.03
GAP-DI/RTV-PDMS	Polydimethylsiloxane	199/1	0.58 ± 0.02	—
GAP-CI/RTV-PDMS	Polydimethylsiloxane	199/1	0.54 ± 0.02	3.08 ± 0.03

AV: acrylic; CI: chemically immobilized; DI- directly incorporated; RTV-PDMS: room-temperature-vulcanizing-polydimethylsiloxane; TZA: triaziridine propionate crosslinker.

The anti-settlement studies with these new coatings (Figure 6) showed that, despite some decreases in larval settlement were observed in DI coatings, the CI GAP in both AV and RTV-PDMS-based formulations showed significant anti-settlement activity ($p < 0.05$), increasing the antifouling performance of both coatings even more, with only 15 and 0% of larvae adhesion being observed after 40 h of exposure, respectively.

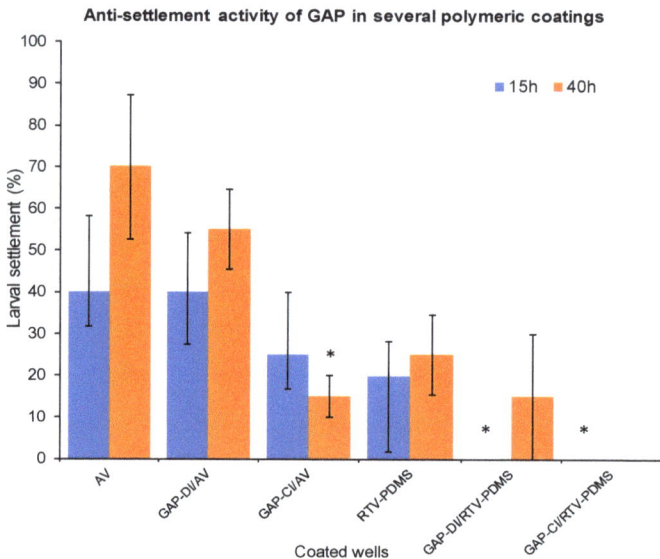

Figure 6. Anti-settlement activity of gallic acid persulfate (GAP) toward the macrofouling organism *Mytilus galloprovincialis larvae* after direct incorporation (DI) and chemical immobilization (CI) in conventional coatings. AV: acrylic; RTV-PDMS: room-temperature-vulcanizing polydimethylsiloxane; h: hours. * Indicates significant differences at $p < 0.05$ (Dunnett test) against the negative controls (AV and RTV-PDMS).

Overall, GAP was responsible for the reduction in the settlement of a problematic marine fouling organism in different polymeric coatings after being chemically immobilized. With this optimized non-release immobilization, this very polar compound might be promising as an environment-friendly alternative resource to replace harmful commercial biocides in AF marine coatings.

3. Materials and Methods

3.1. Materials General Methods

Gallic acid was purchased from Merck (Darmstadt, Germany) (842649); triethylamine sulfur trioxide adduct (T2136) and triethylamine (TO886) were purchased from TCI (Zwijndecht, Belgium) and Sigma-Aldrich (St. Louis, MO, USA), respectively, while TBA-Br, for ion pair chromatography, was purchased from TCI (MFCD00011633, purity > 99.0%), and solvents were purchased from VWR (Radnor, PA, USA), Biosolve (Dieuze, France) and Honeywell (Seelze, Germany). snSW was collected in the Interdisciplinary Centre of Marine and Environmental Research (CIIMAR, Matosinhos, Portugal), treated with a UV filter and filtered using a 0.45-μm syringe filter. ASW was obtained from sera (sera marin salt, Heinsberg, Germany)—33 g/L of sera salt in distilled water.

MW reactions were performed in open glassware vessel reactors in a Milestone Ethos MicroSYNTH 1600 MW (Labstation, ThermoUnicam, Portugal). Thin-layer chromatography (TLC) separations were performed using Merck silica gel 60 (GF254) plates or Macherey–Nagel (Düren, Germany) octadecyl-modified HPTLC silica layers (RP-18 W/UV254). Compounds were visually detected by absorbance at 254 nm and/or 365 nm. Solvents were evaporated using a rotary evaporator under reduced pressure in a Buchi Waterbath B-480 (Flawil, Switzerland). UPW was obtained from the Milli-Q System (Millipore, Darmstadt, Germany).

Infrared spectra for the GAP and GAP–TZA derivative were obtained by FTIR analysis in a Nicolet Magna FTIR 550 Spectrometer coupled with an attenuated total reflectance unit from Smart MiracleTM-Pike Technologies (Fitchurg, WI, USA) with an individual ZnSe crystal. Analyses were performed in the frequency range of 500–4000 cm^{-1} with a 4 cm^{-1} resolution.

^{1}H and ^{13}C (APT) NMR spectra were recorded on a a Bruker Avance 400 spectrometer (Rheinstetten, Germany), operating at 293 K and a frequency of 400.13 MHz for ^{1}H NMR, 100.61 MHz for ^{13}C NMR.

IP-RP-HPLC analyses were performed on a Thermo SCIENTIFIC SpectraSYSTEM (Waltham, MA, USA) equipped with a SpectraSYSTEM UV-8000 diode array detector (DAD), a SpectraSYSTEM P4000 pump and a SpectraSYSTEM AS3000 autosampler, conducted on a Fortis BIO C18 column (Fortis Technologies, 5 µm, 250 × 4.6 mm); the used software was ChromQuest 5.0™.

3.2. Chromatographic Conditions

The mobile phase consisted of acetonitrile:water (62:38 v/v) containing 25 mM of TBA-Br buffer. After mixing, mobile phases were filtered through a 0.45-µm filter and degassed before use by an ultrasonic cleaner (Sonorex Digitec, Bandelin, Berlin, Germany). Chromatographic conditions were set at a constant flow rate of 1 mL/min in isocratic mode, the injection volume was 20 µL, the column was maintained at room temperature (20 ± 2), and the detection wavelength was set a 236 nm. Dissolved snSW GAP was pre-treated before injection, with a dilution of 60 mM of TBA-Br in a proportion of 1:3, allowing us to achieve ion pairing (IP) with a desirable k. This IP-RP-HPLC method was properly developed and validated according the ICH Guidance for Industry Q2 (R1) through several parameters, namely specificity/selectivity, linearity, precision, accuracy, range, limits of detection (LOD) and quantification (LOQ) (Tables S1 and S2) [40]. Concerning the leaching water samples, a different proportion of the mobile phase was used (50:50 v/v), in order to better visualize the signal of GAP without interference.

3.3. Preparation of Standard Solutions

GAP stock solutions from previous synthesis were prepared in UPW and snSW and stored in Eppendorf tubes at −20 °C. Two calibration curves (with three replicates) with the different water types were prepared within the range of 10–500 µM for stability and leaching assays and injected three times into the IP-RP-HPLC system with the UV detector settled at 243 nm. The standard solutions prepared in snSW were diluted with 60 mM of TBA-Br in a proportion of 1:3 prior to injection. A calibration graphic was constructed by plotting the mean peak area versus concentration.

3.4. Water Solubility

The water solubility was evaluated by the Shake Flask method [41]. Briefly, 6 mg of the compound was added to 6 µL of UPW and snSW in Eppendorf tubes. The tube was stirred at 24 ± 1 for 1 h and, after this time, GAP was completely solubilized in both waters. Solubility was defined according to USP [29].

3.5. Stability in Seawater

For the stability assay, 200 µL of stock solution was added to a total of 4 glass vials and each vial was diluted with snSW in order to obtain a final concentration of 200 µM in each vial. After that, 3 of the 4 vials were wrapped in aluminum and stored under different conditions for a period of several months: 1 vial was stored in the refrigerator at a temperature of 4 °C; 1 vial was stored at 18 °C; 1 vial was stored at 24 ± 1; and the other vial was exposed to natural light at 24 ± 1. These procedures were made in duplicate. The same assay was also performed using UPW for comparative purposes.

Periodically, an aliquot of each vial was directly injected into the IP-RP-HPLC system without any extraction procedure, and the peak area of GAP was interpolated into the calibration curve.

3.6. Synthesis of GAP

Gallic acid (Merck 842649, 0.2 g, 1.2 mmoL) was dissolved in DMF (6 mL). Triethylamine (9 eq/OH, 3.30 mL, 32.6 mmoL) and TEA·SO$_3$ (6 eq/OH, 3.8 g, 21.0 mmoL) were added. The mixture was kept under microwave radiation (200 W) at 85–87 °C, for 1 cycle of 1 h. After cooling, the mixture was held at −20 °C overnight. The inferior phase was separated and poured into acetone (100 mL). Triethylamine (12 mL, optimized proportion) was added and the mixture was left at 4 °C for a few hours. The crude oil formed was washed with acetone and ether and dissolved in aqueous solution of 30% sodium acetate (23 mL). Ethanol was added to the suspension to precipitate the sodium salt of the sulfated derivative. The yellow solid yield was 96%. The infrared and NMR data were in accordance with the literature [35]. The purity of GAP was determined by HPLC–DAD analysis with a mobile phase containing an aqueous solution of 25 mM of TBA-Br and acetonitrile (50:50 *v/v*) (>95%, supplementary material Figure S1). The GAP grade used for the several assays was similar (>95%), with a consistent structural characterization.

3.7. Immobilization of GAP in Polymeric Coatings

GAP was immobilized in two main representative biocide-free commercial marine coatings, consisting of two-component systems, a polyurethane (PU)-based system, composed of the base resin F0032 and the curing agent 95580 and a foul-release polydimethylsiloxane (PDMS) system, the HEMPASIL X3 + 87500, composed of the base resin 87509 and the curing agent 98950. Both coating systems were generously provided by Hempel A/S (Copenhagen, Denmark). The immobilization of GAP on those selected marine coating systems followed two strategies, a conventional DI and a CI. For the DI strategy, the GAP agent was first dissolved in *N*-methyl pyrrolidone (NMP, 99.5%, Acros Organics, Geel, Belgium) giving solutions with GAP contents of 18.5 and 15.9 wt.%, which were further added and blended into the paint PU and PDMS components, respectively, and in the exact amounts to yield the desirable GAP contents in the system (c.f. Table 2). The proportions based on the volume of the paint components' bases/curing agents were 2/1 for the PU and 17.8/2.2 for the PDMS wet systems.

For the chemical immobilization strategy, a similar preparation methodology was followed, but with the additional incorporation of a trimethylolpropane triaziridine propionate crosslinker (TZA, 99.5%, PZ Global, Barcelona, Spain), in order to promote the compatibility and the grafting of GAP into the polymeric framework of the coating systems. For this strategy, GAP solutions in NMP at contents of 10.9 and 12.8 wt.% were added and blended in the PU and PDMS-based formulations, respectively. The used base and curing agent proportions for formulation preparation were the ones recommended by the supplier. Finally, the crosslinker was added and blended to the paint system in a content of 2.0 wt.% of the wet formulation.

GAP was also immobilized in two commercial non-marine coatings, an acrylic (AV) (VERKODUR, Ref. 690.195, KORELAX, Trofa, Portugal), and a room-temperature-vulcanizing polydimethylsiloxane, RTV-PDMS (RTV11, MOMENTIVE, Waterford, NY, USA). The immobilization of GAP on those selected coating systems also followed the conventional DI and CI strategies. For the first strategy, the GAP agent was previously dissolved in methyl pyrrolidone (99.5%, Acros Organics, Geel, Belgium), giving a solution containing 11.82 wt.% of GAP, which was further added and blended in the exact amount to provide the GAP-based RTV-PDMS systems (c.f. Table 4). In the case of the acrylic system, the GAP agent was directly added and blended into the acrylic components. The proportions by the volume of the paint components' bases/curing agents were 199/1 and 3/1 for the RTV-PDMS and AV systems, respectively. For the CI strategy, a similar preparation methodology was followed with the additional incorporation of a TZA crosslinker in the blended wet formulation mixture, to promote the compatibility and the grafting of GAP into the respective polymeric matrices.

The optimized GAP contents in the developed polymeric coating formulations and additional additives were chosen in order not to compromise the main final appearance of coating films, such as apparent gloss and adhesion on the substrates used for proof-of-concept in this work, i.e., to accurately coating PVC plates for the 45-day leaching assays and the 24-well microplates for the anti-macrofouling activity assessment.

3.8. Evaluation of the TZA Crosslinker Interaction with GAP

In order to understand the interaction between the crosslinker and the GAP compound applied in the coating formulations to promote the GAP compatibility and its CI, a reaction between GAP and the crosslinker was performed under controlled conditions.

The TZA crosslinker was added to a three-necked round bottom flask, containing GAP (130 mg) dissolved in DMSO (1.15 mL). The mixture, with a GAP/TZA molar ratio of 1.95, was kept at room temperature, under magnetic stirring and an inert atmosphere for 24 h. A precipitate was formed, filtrated and dried in a Buchi R-210/215 rotavapor for FTIR and NMR analysis.

3.9. Leaching Assays

PVC-coated plates (3.5 × 6 cm) with the developed PU and PDMS polymeric coating systems, with or without immobilized GAP, were submerged in ASW for a period of 45 days, using a prior optimized stirring method [36]. The average pH of the ASW during the tests was around 8 ± 0.3, and the temperature ranged from 18 to 21 °C. The obtained leaching water samples were further collected for IP-RP-HPLC analysis.

3.10. Extractive Procedure

Each leaching water was divided in three portions and passed through an OASIS® WAX 6cc cartridge according to the following procedure: the cartridge was conditioned with 6 mL of methanol, followed by 6 mL of water and equilibrated with 6 mL of 25 mM sodium acetate buffer acidified with acetic acid (pH 4); water samples were also acidified with sodium acetate buffer in order to obtain a pH of 4 and then passed through the cartridge; after drying, each cartridge was conditioned with 6 mL of a solution containing methanol and acetonitrile (20:80 v/v) with 2% of ammonium, followed by 2 mL of acetonitrile with 2% of ammonium, and finally 2 mL of acetonitrile; finally, the cartridge was washed with 8 mL of methanol and ammonium (90:10 v/v), followed by 2 mL of methanol basified with ammonium until a pH of 12, and the several solutions were collected in a glass vial. Solvents were reduced to dryness under nitrogen purge by a sample concentrator with a block heater at a temperature of 37 °C. After solvent evaporation, the dried compound was solubilized in 200 µL of UPW, passed through a nylon filter and injected into the IP-RP-HPLC system using a mobile phase containing an aqueous solution with 25 mM of TBA-Br and acetonitrile (50:50 v/v). Recoveries of 100% for this extractive procedure were previously obtained (Figures S8 and S9).

3.11. Anti-Settlement Activity Assessment of GAP Based Coatings

For a preliminary assessment of the behavior/suitability of GAP as bioactive ingredient after its incorporation in coatings, a small-scale laboratory bioassay was developed, based on the bioassay previously used to assess GAP bioactivity against mussel (*Mytilus galloprovincialis*) plantigrades [24]. For this assay, the wells of 24-well microplates were coated with the different GAP formulations to be tested (one formulation per column), and negative control columns were included for each formulation (AF agent-free coating system). The purpose of these bioassays was to determine the ability of the different GAP-based coatings to prevent the fixation of mussel larvae, testing whether the GAP bioactivity towards this macrofouling species is maintained after DI and CI procedures in different coating matrices.

Competent *Mytilus galloprovincialis* plantigrades were collected on Memory Beach (N 41°13′51.5″, W 8°43′15.5″) at low tide, and those showing exploratory behavior were selected in the laboratory and transferred to the coated 24-well microplates. All the coated wells were filled with 2.5 mL snSW (previously treated by UV light and carbon filters and mechanically filtered with 0.45 µM filter before use) to reduce any interferents in relation to mussel larvae fixation ability and health conditions. Each coating, including negative controls, was tested in four replicates (4 wells in a column) with five plantigrades per well in the darkness. After 15 and 40 h, the percentage of larval settlement was determined by the presence/absence of efficiently attached byssal threads, produced by each individual in each condition. The reading times (15 h and 40 h) for larval attachment were selected based on previous trials for bioassay optimization, where 15 h is adequate for maximum thread production and efficient attachment in normal conditions, and 40 h is the maximum time to guarantee the good health status of larvae under bioassay conditions.

3.12. Statistical Analysis

Data from the water stability and anti-settlement screenings were analyzed using a one-way analysis of variance (ANOVA) followed by a Dunnett test against the control ($p < 0.05$). The software IBM SPSS Statistics 21 was used for statistical analysis.

4. Conclusions

In this work, the synthesis of a nature-inspired antifouling compound (GAP) was optimized to maximize GAP production. GAP was obtained with the same purity as the previous methods and with better yields in only 1 h under MW irradiation. This more reproducible, feasible and greener synthesis will certainly allow an easier scale-up synthesis of GAP for future in situ studies and commercialization. MW irradiation is an established way to speed up chemical syntheses, and dominates the pharmaceutical industry, as it improves the homogeneity of the synthesis. Using a parallel scale-up approach, it is possible to achieve scalability for potential industrial adoption by using several vessels simultaneously. Furthermore, it is expected that this technology can increase the overall efficiency of organic synthesis in an environmental friendly way. On the other hand, the obtention of the raw material gallic acid, through the valorization of winery waste by a green extraction method, will also be considered in the future.

Additionally, the several analytical methods developed during this work, using ion pairing chromatography and WAX, provided important contributions to the analysis of sulfated and highly polar compounds in water.

Moreover, the potential of this very polar compound to be applied as an antifouling additive in polymeric coating systems has been proven by its successful immobilization in marine coatings, using a non-leaching strategy promoted by the incorporation of the TZA crosslinker. This triaziridine functional crosslinker reacted with the active hydrogen of the carboxyl function in the GAP structure, thus acting as a bridge molecule between the coating components and GAP. Furthermore, the GAP-based coatings seem to keep their bioactivity, at least regarding the fixation of mussel larvae. These results encourage further in situ studies with GAP as an AF additive in coatings, and an in-depth characterization of the final physical–chemical properties of coatings obtained.

Supplementary Materials: The following are available online at http://www.mdpi.com/1660-3397/18/10/489/s1, Table S1: Linear regression and sensitivity data, Table S2: Accuracy, intra- and inter-day variability (precision), Figure S1: Representative chromatograms of 200 µM of GAP obtained by conventional (green line) and new optimized synthesis (black line), Figure S2: DFT optimized structures of GAP and TZA (ADF/BP86/TZ2P), Figure S3: ^{1}H NMR spectra of gallic acid persulfate (GAP, green line), triaziridine crosslinker (TZA, black line) and GAP–TZA derivative (brown line) in DMSO-d_6 at 293 K, Figure S4: ^{13}C APT NMR spectrum of gallic acid persulfate (GAP) in DMSO-d_6 at 293 K, Figure S5: ^{13}C APT NMR spectrum of triaziridine propionate crosslinker (TZA) in DMSO-d_6 at 293 K, Figure S6: ^{13}C APT NMR spectrum of GAP–TZA derivative in DMSO-d_6 at 293 K, Figure S7: Representative PVC coated plates with commercial marine coatings, from left to right: PU (polyurethane-based control); GAP-CI/PU (PU-based coating containing chemically immobilized (CI) gallic acid persulfate, GAP; PDMS (polydimethylsiloxane-based control); and GAP-CI/PDMS (PDMS-based coating containing CI GAP. Figure S8: Representative chromatograms of 500 µM of GAP dissolved in UPW before and after being passed through the cartridge, Figure S9: Representative chromatograms of 100 µM of GAP dissolved in UPW before and after being passed through the cartridge.

Author Contributions: Conceptualization, E.R.S. and M.C.-d.-S.; data curation, C.V.-B. and F.C.; formal analysis, C.V.-B., S.C. and M.J.C.; funding acquisition, M.C.-d.-S.; investigation, C.V.-B., F.C., B.P., J.R.A. and E.R.S.; methodology, E.S., M.M.M.P., V.V., J.R.A., E.R.S. and M.C.-d.-S.; project administration, M.C.-d.-S. and E.R.S.; resources, M.M.M.P., M.J.C., V.V. and E.R.S.; supervision, J.R.A., E.R.S. and M.C.-d.-S.; validation, C.V.-B. and F.C.; visualization, C.V.-B.; writing—original draft, C.V.-B., J.R.A., E.R.S. and M.C.-d.-S.; writing—review and editing, C.V.-B., E.S., M.M.M.P., M.J.C., V.V., J.R.A., E.R.S. and M.C.-d.-S. All authors have read and agreed to the published version of the manuscript.

Funding: This research was funded by national funds through the Foundation for Science and Technology (FCT) within the scope of research unit grants to CIIMAR (UIDB/04423/2020 and UIDP/04423/2020), to BioISI (UIDB/04046/2020 and UIDP/04046/2020) and under the project PTDC/AAG-TEC/0739/2014 (reference POCI-01-0145-FEDER-016793) supported through national funds provided by FCT and the European Regional Development Fund (ERDF) via the Programa Operacional Factores de Competitividade (POFC/COMPETE) programme and the Reforçar a Investigação, o Desenvolvimento Tecnológico e a Inovação (RIDTI; project 9471).

Acknowledgments: C.V.B. acknowledges FCT for the scholarship SFRH/BD/136147/2018. E.R.S. thanks FCT for her work contract through the Scientific Employment Stimulus—Individual Call—CEECIND/03530/2018.

Conflicts of Interest: The authors declare no conflict of interest.

References

1. Briand, J.-F. Marine antifouling laboratory bioassays: An overview of their diversity. *Biofouling* **2009**, *25*, 297–311. [CrossRef] [PubMed]
2. Holm, E.R. Barnacles and Biofouling. *Integr. Comp. Biol.* **2012**, *52*, 348–355. [CrossRef] [PubMed]
3. Callow, J.A.; Callow, M.E. Trends in the development of environmentally friendly fouling-resistant marine coatings. *Nat. Commun.* **2011**, *2*, 1–10. [CrossRef] [PubMed]
4. Clare, A.S.; Aldred, N. 3—Surface colonisation by marine organisms and its impact on antifouling research. In *Advances in Marine Antifouling Coatings and Technologies*; Hellio, C., Yebra, D., Eds.; Woodhead Publishing: Cambridge, UK, 2009; pp. 46–79.
5. Bixler, G.D.; Bhushan, B. Review article: Biofouling: Lessons from nature. *Philos. Trans. R. Soc. A Math. Phys. Eng. Sci.* **2012**, *370*, 2381–2417. [CrossRef]
6. Demirel, Y.K.; Uzun, D.; Zhang, Y.; Fang, H.-C.; Day, A.H.; Turan, O. Effect of barnacle fouling on ship resistance and powering. *Biofouling* **2017**, *33*, 819–834. [CrossRef]
7. Cao, S.; Wang, J.; Chen, H.; Chen, D. Progress of marine biofouling and antifouling technologies. *Chin. Sci. Bull.* **2011**, *56*, 598–612. [CrossRef]
8. Price, A.R.G.; Readman, J.W.; Gee, D. Booster biocide antifoulants: Is history repeating itself? *Late Lessons Early Warn. Sci. Precaut. Innov.* **2013**, *297*, 265–278.
9. Takahashi, K. Release Rate of Biocides from Antifouling Paints. In *Ecotoxicology of Antifouling Biocides*; Arai, T., Harino, H., Ohji, M., Langston, W.J., Eds.; Springer: Tokyo, Japan, 2009; pp. 3–22.
10. Konstantinou, I.K.; Albanis, T.A. Worldwide occurrence and effects of antifouling paint booster biocides in the aquatic environment: A review. *Environ. Int.* **2004**, *30*, 235–248.
11. Chen, L.; Lam, J.C.W. SeaNine 211 as antifouling biocide: A coastal pollutant of emerging concern. *J. Environ. Sci.* **2017**, *61*, 68–79. [CrossRef]
12. Thomas, K.V.; McHugh, M.; Waldock, M. Antifouling paint booster biocides in UK coastal waters: Inputs, occurrence and environmental fate. *Sci. Total Environ.* **2002**, *293*, 117–127. [CrossRef]
13. Thomas, K.V.; Brooks, S. The environmental fate and effects of antifouling paint biocides. *Biofouling* **2010**, *26*, 73–88. [CrossRef]
14. Martins, S.E.; Fillmann, G.; Lillicrap, A.; Thomas, K.V. Review: Ecotoxicity of organic and organo-metallic antifouling co-biocides and implications for environmental hazard and risk assessments in aquatic ecosystems. *Biofouling* **2018**, *34*, 34–52. [CrossRef] [PubMed]
15. Okamura, H.; Aoyama, I.; Liu, D.; Maguire, R.J.; Pacepavicius, G.J.; Lau, Y.L. Fate and ecotoxicity of the new antifouling compound Irgarol 1051 in the aquatic environment. *Water Res.* **2000**, *34*, 3523–3530. [CrossRef]
16. Silva, E.R.G.; Bordado, J.C.M.; Ferreira, O.R.V. Functionalization Process for Biocide Immobilization in Polymer Matrices. Granted Patent PT108096B (WO2016093719A1), 2019. Available online: https://patents.google.com/patent/PT108096B/en (accessed on 24 September 2020).

17. Silva, E.R.; Ferreira, O.; Ramalho, P.A.; Azevedo, N.F.; Bayón, R.; Igartua, A.; Bordado, J.C.; Calhorda, M.J. Eco-friendly non-biocide-release coatings for marine biofouling prevention. *Sci. Total Environ.* **2019**, *650*, 2499–2511. [CrossRef] [PubMed]
18. Pan, J.; Xie, Q.; Chiang, H.; Peng, Q.; Qian, P.-Y.; Ma, C.; Zhang, G. "From the Nature for the Nature": An Eco-Friendly Antifouling Coating Consisting of Poly(lactic acid)-Based Polyurethane and Natural Antifoulant. *ACS Sustain. Chem. Eng.* **2020**, *8*, 1671–1678. [CrossRef]
19. Ma, C.; Zhang, W.; Zhang, G.; Qian, P.-Y. Environmentally Friendly Antifouling Coatings Based on Biodegradable Polymer and Natural Antifoulant. *ACS Sustain. Chem. Eng.* **2017**, *5*, 6304–6309. [CrossRef]
20. Ciriminna, R.; Bright, F.V.; Pagliaro, M. Ecofriendly Antifouling Marine Coatings. *ACS Sustain. Chem. Eng.* **2015**, *3*, 559–565. [CrossRef]
21. Cui, Y.; Teo, S.; Leong, W.; Chai, C. Searching for "Environmentally-Benign" Antifouling Biocides. *Int. J. Mol. Sci.* **2014**, *15*, 9255. [CrossRef]
22. Vilas-Boas, C.; Sousa, E.; Pinto, M.; Correia-da-Silva, M. An antifouling model from the sea: A review of 25 years of zosteric acid studies. *Biofouling* **2017**, *33*, 927–942. [CrossRef]
23. Carvalhal, F.; Correia-da-Silva, M.; Sousa, E.; Pinto, M.; Kijjoa, A. SULFATION PATHWAYS: Sources and biological activities of marine sulfated steroids. *J. Mol. Endocrinol.* **2018**, *61*, T211. [CrossRef]
24. Almeida, J.; Correia-da-Silva, M.; Sousa, E.; Antunes, J.; Pinto, M.; Vasconcelos, V.; Cunha, I. Antifouling potential of Nature-inspired sulfated compounds. *Sci. Rep.* **2017**, *7*, 42424. [CrossRef] [PubMed]
25. Teixeira, A.; Baenas, N.; Dominguez-Perles, R.; Barros, A.; Rosa, E.; Moreno, D.A.; Garcia-Viguera, C. Natural bioactive compounds from winery by-products as health promoters: A review. *Int. J. Mol. Sci.* **2014**, *15*, 15638–15678. [CrossRef] [PubMed]
26. Species Profile: Mytilus Galloprovincialis. Available online: http://www.iucngisd.org/gisd/species.php?sc=102 (accessed on 31 October 2019).
27. Neves, A.R.; Almeida, J.R.; Carvalhal, F.; Câmara, A.; Pereira, S.; Antunes, J.; Vasconcelos, V.; Pinto, M.; Silva, E.R.; Sousa, E.; et al. Overcoming environmental problems of biocides: Synthetic bile acid derivatives as a sustainable alternative. *Ecotoxicol. Environ. Saf.* **2020**, *187*, 109812. [CrossRef] [PubMed]
28. Wang, X.J.; Tang, Y.H.; Yao, T.W.; Zeng, S. Separation of rutin nona(H-) and deca(H-) sulfonate sodium by ion-pairing reversed-phase liquid chromatography. *J. Chromatogr. A* **2004**, *1036*, 229–232. [CrossRef]
29. USP. *USP Pharmacists' Pharmacopeia*, 2nd ed.; United States Pharmacopeia: Bethesda, MD, USA, 2009; p. S3/13.
30. Correia-da-Silva, M.; Sousa, E.; Duarte, B.; Marques, F.; Carvalho, F.; Cunha-Ribeiro, L.M.; Pinto, M. Polysulfated Xanthones: Multipathway Development of a New Generation of Dual Anticoagulant/Antiplatelet Agents. *J. Med. Chem.* **2011**, *54*, 5373–5384. [CrossRef]
31. Verghese, J.; Liang, A.; Sidhu, P.P.S.; Hindle, M.; Zhou, Q.; Desai, U.R. First steps in the direction of synthetic, allosteric, direct inhibitors of thrombin and factor Xa. *Bioorganic Med. Chem. Lett.* **2009**, *19*, 4126–4129. [CrossRef]
32. Correia-da-Silva, M.; Sousa, E.; Duarte, B.; Marques, F.; Carvalho, F.; Cunha-Ribeiro, L.M.; Pinto, M. Flavonoids with an Oligopolysulfated Moiety: A New Class of Anticoagulant Agents. *J. Med. Chem.* **2011**, *54*, 95–106. [CrossRef]
33. Gill, D.M.; Male, L.; Jones, A.M. Sulfation made simple: A strategy for synthesising sulfated molecules. *Chem. Commun.* **2019**, *55*, 4319–4322. [CrossRef]
34. Ravichandran, S.; Karthikeyan, E. Microwave Synthesis-A Potential Tool for Green Chemistry. *Int. J. ChemTech Res.* **2011**, *3*, 974–4290.
35. Correia-da-Silva, M.; Sousa, E.; Duarte, B.; Marques, F.; Cunha-Ribeiro, L.M.; Pinto, M.M. Dual anticoagulant/antiplatelet persulfated small molecules. *Eur. J. Med. Chem.* **2011**, *46*, 2347–2358. [CrossRef]
36. Ferreira, O.; Rijo, P.; Gomes, J.F.; Santos, R.; Monteiro, S.; Vilas-Boas, C.; Correia-da-Silva, M.; Almada, S.; Alves, L.G.; Bordado, J.C.; et al. Biofouling Inhibition with Grafted Econea Biocide: Toward a Nonreleasing Eco-Friendly Multiresistant Antifouling Coating. *ACS Sustain. Chem. Eng.* **2020**, *8*, 12–17. [CrossRef]
37. Chen, P.-C.; Wang, S.-C.; Huang, C.-Y.; Yeh, J.-T.; Chen, K.-N. New crosslinked polymer from a rapid polymerization of acrylic acid with triaziridine-containing compound. *J. Appl. Polym. Sci.* **2007**, *104*, 809–815.
38. Yebra, D.; Kiil, S.; Dam-Johansen, K. Antifouling technology—Past, present and future steps towards efficient and environmentally friendly antifouling coatings. *Prog. Org. Coat.* **2004**, *50*, 75–104.
39. Zhang, X.M.; Li, L.; Zhang, Y. Study on the Surface Structure and Properties of PDMS/PMMA Antifouling Coatings. *Phys. Procedia* **2013**, *50*, 328–336.

40. ICH. Validation of Analytical Procedures: Text and Methodology. In *Geneva, Q2(R1)*; European Medicines Agency: London, UK, 2005; p. 17.
41. OECD. Guideline for the Testing of Chemicals (Water Solubility). In *N° 105*; Organisation for Economic Co-Operation and Development: Paris, France, 1995.

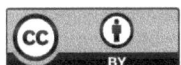

© 2020 by the authors. Licensee MDPI, Basel, Switzerland. This article is an open access article distributed under the terms and conditions of the Creative Commons Attribution (CC BY) license (http://creativecommons.org/licenses/by/4.0/).

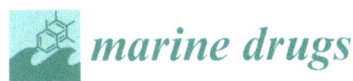

Article

Insights into the Light Response of *Skeletonema marinoi*: Involvement of Ovothiol

Alfonsina Milito [1,2,*], Ida Orefice [3], Arianna Smerilli [3], Immacolata Castellano [1], Alessandra Napolitano [4], Christophe Brunet [3] and Anna Palumbo [1,*]

1. Department of Biology and Evolution of Marine Organisms, Stazione Zoologica Anton Dohrn, Villa Comunale, 80121 Napoli, Italy; immacolata.castellano@szn.it
2. Department of Molecular Genetics, Centre for Research in Agricultural Genomics, Cerdanyola, 08193 Barcelona, Spain
3. Department of Marine Biotechnology, Stazione Zoologica Anton Dohrn, Villa Comunale, 80121 Napoli, Italy; ida.orefice@szn.it (I.O.); arianna.smerilli@szn.it (A.S.); christophe.brunet@szn.it (C.B.)
4. Department of Chemical Sciences, University of Naples "Federico II", 80126 Naples, Italy; alessandra.napolitano@unina.it
* Correspondence: alfonsina.milito@szn.it or alfonsina.milito@cragenomica.es (A.M.); anna.palumbo@szn.it (A.P.); Tel.: +39-081-5833 (ext. 293/276) (A.M.)

Received: 24 July 2020; Accepted: 17 September 2020; Published: 20 September 2020

Abstract: Diatoms are one of the most widespread groups of microalgae on Earth. They possess extraordinary metabolic capabilities, including a great ability to adapt to different light conditions. Recently, we have discovered that the diatom *Skeletonema marinoi* produces the natural antioxidant ovothiol B, until then identified only in clams. In this study, we investigated the light-dependent modulation of ovothiol biosynthesis in *S. marinoi*. Diatoms were exposed to different light conditions, ranging from prolonged darkness to low or high light, also differing in the velocity of intensity increase (sinusoidal *versus* square-wave distribution). The expression of the gene encoding the key ovothiol biosynthetic enzyme, *ovoA*, was upregulated by high sinusoidal light mimicking natural conditions. Under this situation higher levels of reactive oxygen species and nitric oxide as well as ovothiol and glutathione increase were detected. No ovoA modulation was observed under prolonged darkness nor low sinusoidal light. Unnatural conditions such as continuous square-wave light induced a very high oxidative stress leading to a drop in cell growth, without enhancing ovoA gene expression. Only one of the inducible forms of nitric oxide synthase, *nos2*, was upregulated by light with consequent production of NO under sinusoidal light and darkness conditions. Our data suggest that ovothiol biosynthesis is triggered by a combined light stress caused by natural distribution and increased photon flux density, with no influence from the daily light dose. These results open new perspectives for the biotechnological production of ovothiols, which are receiving a great interest for their biological activities in human model systems.

Keywords: algae; antioxidant; diatoms; light; nitric oxide; ovothiol; oxidative stress

1. Introduction

Diatoms represent one of the most widespread and diversified groups of unicellular photosynthetic eukaryotes, widely distributed in all aquatic environments. Due to their relevant abundance in marine ecosystems, they contribute to one-fifth of the photosynthesis carried out on Earth [1] and play a crucial role in biogeochemical cycles [2]. Moreover, diatoms can provide a rich source of bioactive products, including carotenoids, vitamins and polyunsaturated fatty acids [3–5], thus representing promising "biofactories" for biotechnological applications [6,7].

Due to the complex evolutionary history and multiple horizontal gene transfer events from bacteria and viruses [8,9], diatoms possess unique metabolic capabilities, allowing them to adapt to a plethora of ecological niches and to efficiently cope with the environmental forcing variability [10–14]. Among such environmental variables, light is a key factor influencing diatom growth and physiology. Indeed, diatoms are passively transported along the water column, and thus are exposed to very fast changes in light intensity and spectral composition. In a short time frame, the same species can switch from darkness or a very low light intensity environment—with dominance of blue and/or green as well as absence of red wavelength—to very high light intensity characterized by the full range of visible wavelengths (400–700 nm) [14]. Diatoms evolved an efficient ability to adapt to different light conditions by modulating the levels of photosynthetic and photoprotective pigments, as well as of antioxidant compounds, especially carotenoids [15–19]. Among carotenoids, pigments forming the xanthophyll cycle (XC) are responsible for most of the short-term photoprotection, including the non-photochemical quenching of chlorophyll α fluorescence (NPQ) [18,20–22]. High light intensity, or more generally light induced stress, also promotes the synthesis of other antioxidants, such as ascorbic and phenolic acid, as well as the activation of antioxidant enzymes [18,19].

Recently, we have discovered that the coastal centric diatom *Skeletonema marinoi*, grown under moderate light condition, produces micromolar concentrations of ovothiol B [23], hitherto identified only in clams [24].

Ovothiol B belongs to the π-methyl-5-thiohistidines class (ovothiols), considered powerful antioxidants and mainly found in marine invertebrates, proteobacteria and protists, e.g., microalgae [25]. Due to the aromaticity of the imidazole ring, ovothiols possess a highly acidic thiol group (pKa = 1.4) compared to other cellular thiols, such as glutathione (pKa = 8.75) [26–28]. This chemical feature is related to the ability of ovothiols to act as efficient scavengers of radicals and peroxides [29]. Ovothiols have been receiving great interest for their biological activities in *in vitro* and *in vivo* human model systems. Indeed, they exhibited pleiotropic beneficial properties, revealing antifibrotic activities in a murine model of liver fibrosis [30,31], antiproliferative action in human cancer cell lines [32–34] and anti-inflammatory effects in endothelial cells derived from women affected by gestational diabetes [35]. Ovothiols are synthesized *in vivo* by two key enzymes, the sulfoxide synthase OvoA and the β-lyase OvoB [36,37], in three different forms, A, B and C, differing in the methylation state of the α-amino group. Ovothiol B is a monomethylated form, while ovothiol A lacks this methyl and ovothiol C possesses two methyl groups [25].

Only few studies performed on microalgae have highlighted some connections between ovothiol biosynthesis and light-dependent processes. Indeed, ovothiol was reported to be a redox regulator, controlling the activity of the chloroplast-coupling factor in *Dunaliella salina* [38]. Moreover, different ovoA transcripts were identified in *Euglena gracilis* under dark or sunlight conditions [39].

The present study is intended to explore more systematically the possible role of ovothiol in the light-dependent response of the diatom *S. marinoi* and to understand if this poorly known antioxidant could contribute to defend diatoms from light stress. To this aim, *S. marinoi* cells were exposed to different light regimes, varying in photon flux density (PFD), velocity of intensity increase (sinusoidal *versus* square-wave distribution) and light:dark photoperiod cycle. We tested the hypothesis that changes in light conditions could affect the expression of the gene *ovoA* encoding the key ovothiol biosynthetic enzyme. Moreover, to investigate whether ovothiol biosynthesis may be part of the cellular antioxidant response, we monitored the cellular stress status by measuring the concentration of reactive oxygen species (ROS) and nitric oxide (NO), important messengers of stress response [40–43], as well as the expression of the enzyme responsible for NO biosynthesis, e.g., NO synthase, recently identified in diatoms [44]. We also tested the possibility that light-induced upregulation of *ovoA* gene expression could result in an increased ovothiol production, activating the complete biosynthetic machinery necessary for its biosynthesis. The outcomes of the present work open new perspectives on the possible exploitation of diatoms for a large-scale production of this compound. Indeed, diatoms' biomass enriched with antioxidant molecules (ovothiol, carotenoids, polyphenols, etc.) may represent an ecofriendly solution for biotechnological purposes, especially using light as a manipulating factor [45].

2. Results

2.1. Molecular Response to High Light Conditions

We evaluated the molecular response of the diatom *Skeletonema marinoi* under a moderate light condition, used as a non-stressful control (low sinusoidal light, having midday light intensity peak at 150 µmol photons s^{-1} m^{-2}, Sin150), as well as under high light stressful conditions, including high sinusoidal light peaking at 600 µmol photons s^{-1} m^{-2} (Sin600), high square-wave light peaking at 300 (Square300) and 600 µmol photons s^{-1} m^{-2} (Square600). These light conditions vary in both light intensity distribution over time (sinusoidal *vs.* square-wave), in the midday light intensity peak (150 *vs.* 300 *vs.* 600 µmol photons s^{-1} m^{-2}) and in the daily light dose (3.6 mol photons m^{-2} d^{-1} for Sin150, 14.4 mol photons m^{-2} d^{-1} for Sin600 and Square300, 28.8 mol photons m^{-2} d^{-1} for Square600).

Under the different experimental conditions, we assessed the expression of *ovoA* and *nos* genes to highlight their eventual light modulation at different time points. Samples were taken at 0, 6 and 24 h under all conditions, while additional samples were included in the high stressful light conditions. An earlier time point (2 h) was taken under Sin600 and two additional samplings (0.2 and 2 h) were carried out under Square300 and Square600 conditions, to evaluate the early response under high light stress. In *S. marinoi* two nos transcripts have been previously identified but no data are available on their functional significance [44]. Interestingly, our *in silico* analysis showed that both *S. marinoi* Nos protein sequences lack the inhibitory loop (Supplementary Figure S1), which is a feature of inducible Nos, making it Ca^{2+}-independent [46]. To detect the redox status of the cells, in all experimental conditions we also measured the levels of reactive oxygen species (ROS) and nitric oxide (NO) through biochemical assays.

Under the control light condition (Sin150), no modulation of *ovoA* expression was observed at any experimental time both in exponential and in stationary growth phases (Figure 1A). The same was observed for *nos1* and *nos2*, except for a *nos1* down-regulation at the midday light intensity peak in exponential growth phase (6 h), with a decreasing trend also at the midday peak in the stationary phase (30 h, Figure 1A). Both NO and ROS levels were higher in stationary compared to the exponential growth phase, while they did not vary during the day in the exponential growth phase, confirming the non-stressful nature of this control condition (Figure 1A). Cultures exposed to Sin600 showed an upregulation of *ovoA* gene expression after 2 and 6 h from the light switch (Figure 1B). Additionally, *nos2* upregulation was observed after 6 h, while no variation was observed for *nos1* (Figure 1B). Both NO and ROS levels increased at 6 h and 24 h from light switch to Sin600 (Figure 1B).

To investigate whether the *ovoA* gene upregulation observed at 6 h of Sin600, compared to Sin150, resulted also in increased production of the molecule, we measured the concentration of ovothiol both under Sin600 and Sin150, at the midday light intensity peaks 600 and 150 µmol photons s^{-1} m^{-2}, respectively. We also evaluated the content of the other major intracellular thiol glutathione. In agreement with the upregulation of *ovoA*, the cellular content of ovothiol B increased by two-fold from 50 µM under Sin150 to 110 µM under Sin600 (Figure 1A; Table 1). Similarly, glutathione also doubled its concentration from 1 mM under control condition (Sin150) to 2.3 mM under high sinusoidal light (Sin600; Table 1).

Cells moved to Square300 did not show any significant modulation in the expression of *ovoA* nor of *nos*, neither at a very early time point (0.2 h). The concentrations of NO and ROS did not increase, with the exception of a significant ROS overproduction at 24 h, following the night phase (Figure 2A). Similarly, no gene modulation was observed in the Square600 condition, at any experimental time, with ROS significantly increasing at 24 h (Figure 2B).

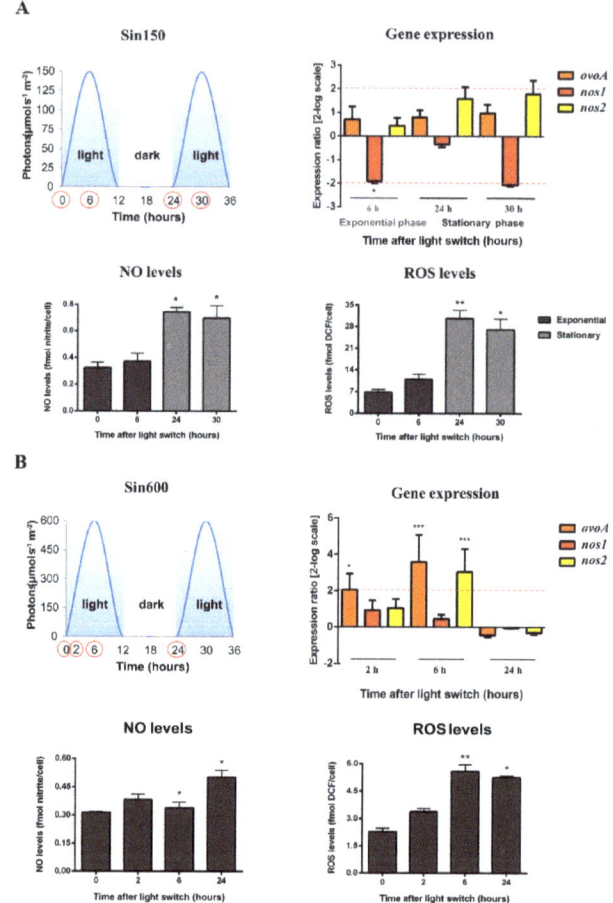

Figure 1. *S. marinoi* under control and high sinusoidal light conditions. Scatter plot representing light condition, gene expression data, NO and ROS levels were reported. (**A**) Control condition with midday peak at 150 µmol photons s^{-1} m^{-2} (low sinusoidal light, Sin150); (**B**) High sinusoidal light with midday peak at 600 µmol photons s^{-1} m^{-2} (Sin600). The light:dark photoperiod cycle was 12 h:12 h. Sampling times were highlighted in the light scatter plot by red circles. Fold gene expression data were analyzed by the pairwise fixed reallocation randomization test by REST and are here reported as 2-log scale mean ± standard error and. NO and ROS data were analyzed by Kruskal–Wallis with a Dunn's post hoc test and are reported as mean ± standard deviation. * $p < 0.05$, ** $p < 0.01$ and *** $p < 0.001$ represent significance compared to 0 time.

Table 1. Thiols determination in *S. marinoi*. The concentrations of ovothiol B and glutathione in *S. marinoi* under control (Sin150) and high sinusoidal (Sin600) light conditions are reported as mean ± standard deviation.

Light Condition	Ovothiol B Concentration	Glutathione Concentration
Low sinusoidal light (Sin150)	50 ± 10 µM	1.0 ± 0.3 mM
High sinusoidal light (Sin600)	110 ± 20 µM	2.3 ± 0.3 mM

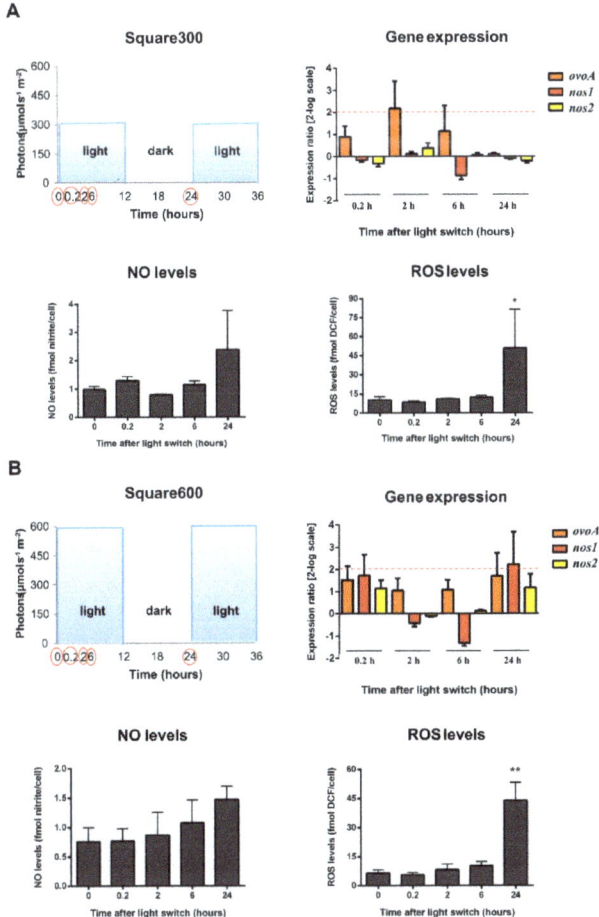

Figure 2. *S. marinoi* under high square-wave light conditions. Scatter plot representing light condition, gene expression data, NO and ROS levels were reported. (**A**) High square-wave light with midday peak at 300 µmol photons s^{-1} m^{-2} (Square300); (**B**) High square-wave light with midday peak at 600 µmol photons s^{-1} m^{-2} (Square600). The light:dark photoperiod cycle was 12 h:12 h. Sampling times were highlighted in the light scatter plot by red circles. Fold gene expression data were analyzed by the pairwise fixed reallocation randomization test by REST and are here reported as 2-log scale mean ± standard error and. NO and ROS data were analyzed by Kruskal–Wallis with a Dunn's post hoc test and are reported as mean ± standard deviation. * $p < 0.05$ and ** $p < 0.01$ represent significance compared to 0 time.

Interestingly, cells under both square-wave lights (Square300 and Square600) displayed a very high oxidative stress at 24 h, following the night phase (ROS content about 45 fmol DCF/cell; Figure 2A,B), compared to cells under Sin600 (ROS content about 5 fmol DCF/cell; Figure 1B). Indeed, this latter condition, although being characterized by a high intensity of light, mimics a natural climate, progressively increasing the light intensity until the midday peak. Conversely, under the square-wave distribution, cells are suddenly exposed to the maximal light intensity, not allowing the acclimation process, which occurs in natural conditions. The detrimental effect of the square-wave light conditions

2.2. Molecular Response to Prolonged Darkness and Low Light Conditions

In a next step, we assessed the molecular response to prolonged darkness (0 h:24 h light:dark photoperiod cycle) and very low light conditions (midday light intensity peak at 10 µmol photons s^{-1} m^{-2}), i.e., Sin10 and Square10, varying in both light:dark photoperiod cycles (12 h:12 h and 24 h:0 h, respectively) and in light distribution over time (sinusoidal vs. square-wave, respectively). In these conditions, samplings were carried out at dawn and midday peak of two consecutive days (0, 6, 24 and 30 h) to follow two consecutive light:dark photoperiod cycles.

Cells exposed to a continuous dark condition showed a significant *nos2* upregulation after 24 h without any *ovoA* modulation (Figure 3). NO levels increased at 24 h, while the concentration of ROS was upregulated at 30 h (Figure 3).

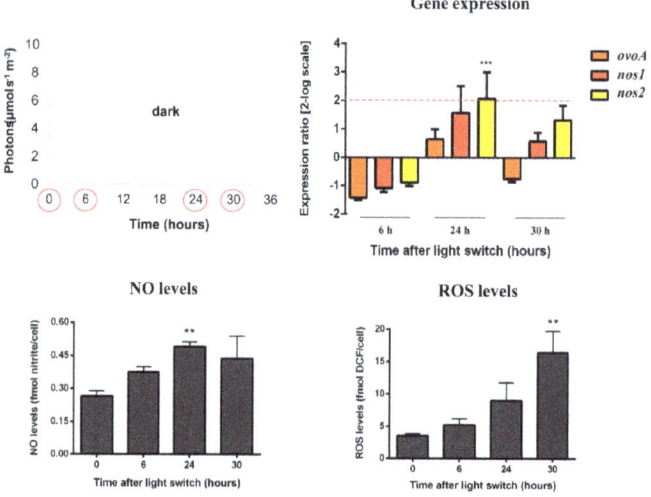

Figure 3. *S. marinoi* under dark condition. Scatter plot representing the dark condition, gene expression data, NO and ROS levels were reported. Dark was kept constant for all the experiment (light:dark photoperiod cycle 0 h:24 h). Sampling times were highlighted in the scatter plot by red circles. Fold gene expression data were analyzed by the pairwise fixed reallocation randomization test by REST and are here reported as 2-log scale mean ± standard error and. NO and ROS data were analyzed by Kruskal–Wallis with a Dunn's post hoc test and are reported as mean ± standard deviation. ** $p < 0.01$ and *** $p < 0.001$ represent significance compared to 0 time.

Cells shifted to Sin10 did not modulate *ovoA* nor *nos1* gene expression, while *nos2* was upregulated after 24 h from the light switch (Figure 4A). NO and ROS variations under Sin10 condition resembled the pattern obtained under prolonged darkness. Indeed, levels increased after 24 h and 30 h, for NO and ROS respectively (Figure 4A).

Under continuous Square10 condition, *nos1* was downregulated after 24 h from the light switch, while all the target genes were significantly downregulated at 30 h. In parallel, NO and ROS increased levels were observed at the same times, with ROS reaching very high concentrations (about 100–150 fmol DCF/cell, Figure 4B).

Among these three conditions, Square10 resulted to be the most stressful for the cells, as also highlighted by the drop in cell growth observed at 24 h (Supplementary Table S1).

Pairwise Pearson correlation analyses were performed between the different variables in three clusters of light conditions: low light (Sin150, Sin10 and Square10), high light (Sin600, Square300 and Square600) and dark. In the high light cluster, *ovoA* was correlated to *nos2*, and ROS levels were positively correlated to NO and *nos1* (Table 2). Similarly, under low light NO was correlated with ROS while *ovoA* with both *nos1* and *nos2*, and *nos1* with *nos2* (Table 2). In the dark condition, only NO-*ovoA* and ROS-*nos1* pairs were correlated (Table 2). These results displayed the different pattern and potential interactions between these variables shaped by the light quantity harvested by cells.

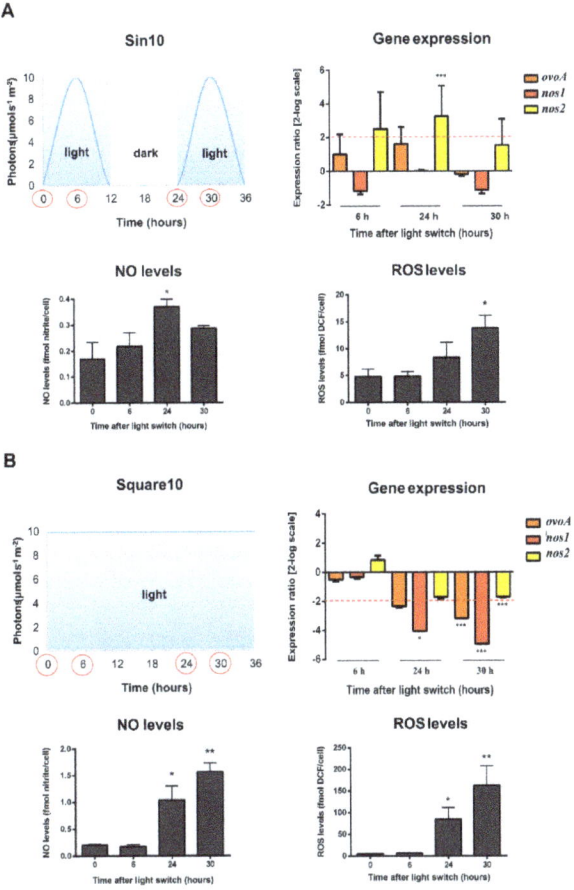

Figure 4. *S. marinoi* under very low sinusoidal and square-wave light conditions. Scatter plot representing light condition, gene expression data, NO and ROS levels were reported. (**A**) Very low sinusoidal light with a midday peak at 10 µmol photons s^{-1} m^{-2} (Sin10). The light:dark photoperiod cycle was 12 h:12 h; (**B**) Very low square-wave light was kept constant for all the experiment at 10 µmol photons s^{-1} m^{-2} (Square 10). The light:dark photoperiod cycle was 24 h:0 h. Sampling times were highlighted in the light scatter plot by red circles. Fold gene expression data were analyzed by the pairwise fixed reallocation randomization test by REST and are here reported as 2-log scale mean ± standard error and. NO and ROS data were analyzed by Kruskal–Wallis with a Dunn's post hoc test and are reported as mean ± standard deviation. * $p < 0.05$, ** $p < 0.01$ and *** $p < 0.001$ represent significance compared to time 0.

Table 2. Pairwise Pearson correlation analyses conducted on all variables (fold gene expression ratios, NO and ROS levels). Different colors refer to different light conditions (red = high light (HL), blue = low light (LL) and green = dark (D)). HL, LL and D indicate the light intensity at which the indicated pair is positively correlated. * $p < 0.05$, ** $p < 0.01$ and *** $p < 0.001$ represent significance of positive correlation.

	NO	ROS	ovoA	nos1	nos2
NO		HL, LL	D	-	-
EOS	*** $p < 0.001$, *** $p < 0.001$		-	HL, D	-
ovoA	* $p < 0.05$	-		LL	HL, LL
nos1	-	* $p < 0.05$, * $p < 0.05$	** $p < 0.01$		LL
nos2	-	-	*** $p < 0.001$, *** $p < 0.001$	** $p < 0.01$	

3. Discussion

Ovothiols are natural sulfur compounds mainly occurring in marine organisms and in the microbial world, in three differentially methylated forms: A, B and C [25]. The biological role of these molecules has often been linked to their peculiar antioxidant properties [26,27] mediating defense from oxidative stress during fertilization and development in the sea urchin [47,48], from environmental stressors in fish eye lenses [49], from macrophage-triggered stress in pathogenic parasites during infection [50] and from light-dependent stress in microalgae [38,39]. In addition, ovothiols have been recently suggested to protect the sea anemone from the stress induced by UV radiation [51] and mussels from environmental pollutants during spawning [52]. However, biological functions not strictly related to oxidative stress have also been discovered. For example, ovothiols have been reported to induce egg release in marine polychaetes during sexual reproduction [53]. Interestingly, ovothiols might play important roles also in animals that, although lacking the biosynthetic pathway, might acquire this bioactive compound from external sources [49,54,55].

We recently described the occurrence and distribution of OvoA in diatoms and we identified ovothiol B as the ovothiol form produced by the coastal centric diatom *Skeletonema marinoi* at micromolar concentrations, when grown under moderate light condition [23]. Our hypothesis is that ovothiol biosynthesis could have been evolved and conserved in diatoms to help them to defend from the oxidative stress enhanced by high light, thus contributing to the ecological success of these photosynthetic protists. Following this assumption, we investigated the light-dependent regulation of ovothiol B biosynthesis in *S. marinoi*, mainly examining the expression of the gene *ovoA* encoding the key ovothiol biosynthetic enzyme.

The experimental strategy adopted in this study involved the cultivation of *S. marinoi* cells under different stressful light conditions, following a preacclimation period under moderate light. For each condition, samples were collected at different time points and were analyzed for gene expression of *ovoA* as well as for intracellular concentration of reactive oxygen species (ROS) and nitric oxide (NO), considered key mediators of stress response [11,40–43,56]. To integrate data on NO production and to investigate a possible involvement of the arginine-dependent NO biosynthesis in response to stressful light conditions, we also followed the gene expression of NO synthases in *S. marinoi*, which we named *nos1* and *nos2*. Among all the conditions tested, the high sinusoidal light (Sin600) resulted to be the most efficient in inducing an increased expression of *ovoA*. Indeed, *ovoA* is upregulated after only 2 and 6 h from the light switch with a significant increase in NO and ROS content at 6 h, as well as ovothiol production, which doubles its concentration compared to the control condition. Under this light, also *nos2* is upregulated after 6 h from a light switch together with increased NO levels already at 6 h and maintained high until 24 h, while *nos1* is not modulated at any experimental time. This may indicate a different role for these two nos transcripts. The *in silico* analysis of the Nos1/2 protein primary structure points out an inducible nature of the two Nos isoforms, but our data suggest that only Nos2 responds to high light, with a concomitant increase of NO. This issue is quite interesting and would deserve further investigation to understand which factors may be involved in Nos1 induction.

The finding that *ovoA* is not modulated in cells under square-wave light conditions suggests that the exposure to fast increases in photon flux density (PFD) does not allow the cells to efficiently modulate their metabolism, as also evident from the very high oxidative stress observed in cells at 24 h from the light switch to Square300 and Square600. Indeed, these unnatural conditions likely compromise the physiological defense mechanisms, finally leading to cell death, as indicated by the observed drop in cell growth. Even at a very early time (0.2 h) the cells do not exhibit any response in terms of *ovoA* modulation and other measured variables. Interestingly, our data are in line with a recent study evaluating the overall response of *S. marinoi* to different light regimes in terms of activated photoprotective and antioxidant systems, including ascorbic acid, one of the most abundant intracellular antioxidants, carotenoids and phenolic compounds, which significantly increase under the Sin600 condition [19]. Thus, the finding that both ovothiol and glutathione double their content in Sin600 condition may indicate that this light regime is able to modulate the diatom metabolism such that all the triggered photoprotective and antioxidant systems may synergically contribute to the defense from the high light stress. Indeed, the increased ovothiol production under the Sin600 condition suggests that this condition not only induces OvoA activity but also all the enzymatic toolkit necessary for ovothiol B biosynthesis, including the lyase OvoB and the still uncharacterized methyltransferase [36,37,55]. Moreover, the uncommon antioxidant properties of ovothiols compared to other thiols, including glutathione [26–28], can partially explain the observed difference in concentration of these two thiols in *S. marinoi*, suggesting that very low levels of ovothiol could be enough to exploit its antioxidant function.

The lack of *ovoA* modulation in Square300 highlights that the daily light dose is not a trigger for the increase of *ovoA* expression, since this condition is characterized by the same daily light dose as Sin600 (around 14.4 mol photons m^{-2} for both Sin600 and Square300), which is conversely able to stimulate ovothiol biosynthesis. Moreover, ovothiol biosynthesis does not react to fast increases of PFD, provided with Square600 condition, but instead to a gradual PFD increase under Sin600 condition.

These results highlight the phenotypic plasticity of *S. marinoi* when submitted to different light conditions, with ovothiol involvement into the photoresponse when cells cope with natural high light condition (sinusoidal), while it does not take part to the response of cells to unnatural high light condition. This is a quite interesting issue being that phenotypic plasticity, defined as the ability of an organism's genotype to display different phenotypes in response to the environmental variability, is a key process explaining microalgal adaptability to natural conditions [57–59]. In particular, microalgae are adapted to a natural light sinusoidal distribution during the day, allowing them to efficiently cope with light variations, e.g., high light environment, through the activation of different kinds of complementary photoresponses, from the fast non-photochemical quenching or xanthophyll cycle operation to changes in carotenoids levels or in antioxidant network activation. When cells are submitted to unnatural light variations (e.g., square-wave distribution or very fast light increase), they undergo physiological/biochemical stress responses, which are different in amplitude and time succession sequence compared to responses to natural light conditions [16–19,60].

The results of our study let us hypothesize that ovothiol synthesis/activation is among the players into the natural physiological response of microalgae to high light, but seems not to be a way for cells to cope with highly stressful (unnatural) light conditions. This might be due to the high-energy cost for cells to synthesize ovothiol, or, more likely, to the lack of biological intracellular signal for the activation of ovothiol biosynthesis.

Yet, the lack of *ovoA* modulation during the stationary growth phase reinforces the finding that the transcriptional level of *ovoA* responds to light and is not modulated by other physiological stressful processes, such as senescence.

The results on *ovoA* modulation under darkness and very low light conditions confirm the key role of light in enhancing ovothiol biosynthesis. Indeed, while there is basically no *ovoA* modulation under prolonged darkness and Sin10 condition (12 h:12 h light:dark), cells grown under continuous Square10 (24 h:0 h light:dark) display a downregulation of the genes *ovoA* and *nos1/2* over time, reaching a high significance at 30 h from the light switch, together with an increase of NO and ROS levels, and a drastic decrease in cell growth rate. This may be due to the extremely unnatural character of this condition. By contrast, diatoms can tolerate prolonged darkness and very low sinusoidal light, since they naturally experience these conditions when they sink at the limit or below the photic zone. These results may indicate that the absence of *ovoA* upregulation under darkness and low light conditions leads to very low levels of ovothiol, which are presumably not enough to counteract the enhanced oxidative stress. Interestingly also other antioxidants and protective systems do not increase in dark and low light conditions, thus underlining a crucial role of light to induce the production of photoprotective and antioxidant systems, excluding an internal circadian clock [19].

Overall, the conditions mostly affecting the variables here measured are Sin600 and Square10. Indeed, while a too high intensity light could damage the photosynthetic apparatus of diatoms, also a prolonged light, even though at very low light intensity, could cause a chronic accumulation of ROS and lead to cell death, as observed. However, the upregulation of antioxidant systems, including ovothiol biosynthesis, by high sinusoidal light allows the cells to better tolerate the stress, while cells experiencing a low light (or dark) stress are not able to efficiently respond due to the absence of light modulation of such defense systems.

The present work might provide the basis for a possible eco-sustainable production of ovothiols by diatoms, to be used as "biofactories" for biotechnological purposes through the light modulation of their growth, metabolism and physiology [3,7,19,61–63]. Indeed, despite the increasing interest in the pharmaceutical potential of this class of molecules endowed with antiproliferative, anti-inflammatory and antifibrotic properties [30–35], studies regarding their bioactivities are still limited by the small amounts of ovothiol available for applied research. Currently, they can be extracted by sea urchin eggs, thus obtaining 2.5 mg of pure ovothiol A from 10 g of wet material [25,32]. However, sea urchins cannot provide sufficient amounts of ovothiols for extensive studies, also considering the necessity to preserve natural populations at sea. On the other hand, the light-induced upregulation of ovothiol formation by 2-fold might still be not enough to allow an efficient exploitation of such system for biotechnological purposes. Therefore, further studies will be necessary to find alternative and more efficient growth conditions, e.g., different nutrient availabilities, that might be able to increase ovothiol levels more efficiently, or genetic engineering of diatoms to optimize the ovothiol biosynthesis by gene manipulation.

4. Materials and Methods

4.1. Experimental Strategy and Sampling

The coastal centric diatom *Skeletonema marinoi* Sarno and Zingone (strain CCMP 2092) was used as the model species in this work for its high growth rate [16,64] and its use in aquaculture and biotechnology [18,19,65–68]. Additionally, the biology and photophysiology of this species are well known [16,63]. The strain (CCMP 2092) used in this work was collected from surface waters of the Northern Adriatic Sea, where this diatom provides the major contribution to the late winter blooms [69]. *S. marinoi* cultures were carried out in 4.5 L glass flasks under water movement, provided by an aquarium wave maker pump (Sunsun, JVP-110) at 20 °C, containing seawater previously prefiltered through a 0.7 µm GF/F glass-fiber filter (Whatman™) autoclaved and enriched with F/2 medium nutrients [70] with some modifications. In particular, to ensure enough nutrient supply, the content of essential nutrients (phosphate, dissolved silica, trace metals and vitamins) in the culture medium was doubled [63]. Light was provided by a custom-built LED illumination system, able to modulate light intensity and spectral composition (Patent number: EP 13196793.7) [14]. Light intensity was measured inside each flask by using a laboratory PAR4π sensor (QSL 2101, Biospherical Instruments Inc., San Diego, CA, USA). The light spectral composition was kept constant during the preacclimation and all the experimental conditions were set up with a ratio blue:green:red = 50:40:10, usually found in the first layers of the photic zone at sea [14]. Preacclimation of cells was performed for a minimum of two weeks at a moderate light intensity, 12 h:12 h light:dark photoperiod, with a sinusoidal intensity distribution peaking at 150 µmol photons s^{-1} m^{-2} after 6 h from dawn (Sin150). Each experiment included three independent cultures and lasted 1–2 days, after the shift from the preacclimation condition to the experimental light condition. Both sinusoidal and square-wave light distributions were applied at different intensities in order to investigate the effect of different velocities of light increase on ovothiol biosynthesis [60]. Sinusoidal distribution is similar to the natural condition, with a succession of dawn, gradual light increase up to the midday intensity peak and gradual light decrease up to sunset. By contrast, the square-wave distribution—generally used in indoor algal cultivation systems—constitutes an unnatural condition, providing a fast increase of light intensity, kept constant for all the day phase (12 h) and then switched off for the night phase (12 h).

The seven experimental conditions were:

- Darkness (continuous absence of light; 0 h:24 h light:dark; daily light dose: 0 mol photons m^{-2});
- Very low sinusoidal light 10 (midday light intensity peak: 10 µmol photons s^{-1} m^{-2}; 12 h:12 h light:dark; daily light dose: 0.24 mol photons m^{-2}; Sin10);
- Very low square-wave light 10 (continuous light intensity: 10 µmol photons s^{-1} m^{-2}; 24 h:0 h light:dark; daily light dose: 1 mol photons m^{-2}; Square10);
- Low sinusoidal light 150 (midday light intensity peak: 150 µmol photons s^{-1} m^{-2}; 12 h:12 h light:dark; daily light dose: 3.6 mol photons m^{-2}; Sin150);
- High sinusoidal light 600 (midday light intensity peak: 600 µmol photons s^{-1} m^{-2}; 12 h:12 h light:dark; daily light dose: 14.4 mol photons m^{-2}; Sin600);
- High square-wave light 300 (continuous light intensity: 300 µmol photons s^{-1} m^{-2}; 12 h:12 h light:dark; daily light dose: 14.4 mol photons m^{-2}; Square300);
- High square-wave light 600 (continuous light intensity: 600 µmol photons s^{-1} m^{-2}; 12 h:12 h light:dark; daily light dose: 28.8 mol photons m^{-2}; Square600).

The Square300 condition provided the same daily light dose experienced by cells grown under Sin600, allowing us to compare square-wave and sinusoidal distributions of light, without any influence from different daily light doses [19]. All experimental conditions provided a 12 h:12 h light:dark photoperiod except for the conditions Square10 (very low intensity light was kept constant for all the duration of the experiment) and darkness (no "day phase" for all the duration of the experiment).

For each experimental condition, samplings were performed in the exponential growth phase, except for the control light condition (Sin150) in which samplings were done both in exponential and stationary growth phases.

In particular, for all the conditions samples were taken at predawn (time 0 h), at 6 h (midday peak) and 24 h (at the end of the night phase) from the light switch. Since high light is known to trigger rapid photoprotective processes in phytoplankton species [71] an additional sampling at 2 h was performed for Sin600, Square300 and Square600. In case of the square-wave light conditions (Square300 and Square600), in which cells experienced a very unnatural and fast increase of light intensity, samples were taken also at 0.2 h (12 min) to evaluate the short-term response. In case of very low sinusoidal and square-wave lights and darkness conditions, in which cells experienced different light:dark photoperiod cycles, samplings were done at 0 and 6 h for two consecutive days.

4.2. Cell Density

Cell density was monitored during the experiments to obtain growth curves. Briefly, 2 mL subsamples from each flask were collected and fixed with Lugol's iodine solution (1.5% *v/v*). One milliliter of this solution was used to fill a Sedgewick Rafter counting cell chamber and cell counts were performed by using a Zeiss Axioskop 2 Plus light microscope (Carl Zeiss, Göttingen, Germany).

4.3. RNA Extraction, Reverse Transcription and Best Reference Genes Assessment

Diatom samples (50 mL) were collected at different times from dawn by centrifugation at 3200 rcf for 30 min at 4 °C. The final pellets were resuspended in 800 µL TRIZOL, frozen in liquid nitrogen and stored at −80 °C until use. The total RNA was extracted according to Barra et al., 2013 [41] and subjected to DNase treatment using DNase I recombinant, RNase-free (Roche, Basel, Switzerland), according to the manufacturer's protocol. RNeasy MinElute Cleanup Kit (Qiagen, Venlo, The Netherlands) was used to purify and concentrate the total RNA, finally eluted in 20 µL RNase-free water. RNA samples were quantified by assessing the absorbance at 260 nm (ND-1000 Spectrophotometer; NanoDrop Technologies, Wilmington, DE, USA.) and then checked for integrity by agarose gel electrophoresis. Possible gDNA contamination was checked by PCR on RNA samples and agarose gel electrophoresis. From each RNA sample 1 µg was retrotranscribed in complementary DNA (cDNA) using the iScriptTM cDNA synthesis kit (Bio-Rad Laboratories, Hercules, CA, USA) and the T100 Thermal cycler (Bio-Rad Laboratories, Hercules, CA, USA), following the manufacturer's instructions. In order to analyze the expression levels of target genes, five putative reference genes were analyzed by RT-qPCR to find the most stable genes in our conditions. The selected genes were histone 4 (*H4*), α- tubulin (*TUB A*), elongation factor 1α (*EF1α*), glyceraldehyde-3-phosphate dehydrogenase (*GAPDH*) and actin (*ACT*). For the amplification of putative reference genes, specific primers reported in the literature were used [72]. The best reference gene for each condition was identified by crossing results obtained with two different algorithms: BestKeeper [73] and NormFinder [74]. In particular, *H4* was used as a reference gene in the following conditions: Sin600, Square300 and darkness; *GADPH* was used for Square10; *ACT* for Square600 and *TUB A* for Sin10 and Sin150.

4.4. Reverse Transcription-Quantitative PCR (RT-qPCR) Experiments

For *ovoA*, the expression levels of the transcript SmOvoA_2388 containing all the canonical domains of metazoan OvoAs [23] were examined. For *nos* genes, the expression of two different transcripts previously reported in *S. marinoi* [44] was analyzed. We named the two *nos* genes: *nos1* and *nos2* (for details see Materials and Methods 4.8.). Specific primers were designed using Primer3 program V. 4.1.0 (primer3.ut.ee) considering the putative sequences reported in the *S. marinoi* transcriptome (MMETSP1039, http://datacommons.cyverse.org/browse/iplant/home/shared/imicrobe/camera/camera_mmetsp_ncgr). RT-qPCR was performed in a MicroAmp Optical 384-Well reaction plate (Applied Biosystems, Foster City, CA, USA) with optical adhesive covers in a Viia7 Real Time PCR System (Applied Biosystem, Foster City, CA, USA). The oligos used to amplify the target genes were reported in Table S2. Serial dilutions of cDNA and the obtained cycle (Ct) mean values were used to generate the standard curves in order to calculate primer reaction efficiency (E= $10^{-1/\text{slope}}$) and correlation factor R2 (Table S2). The RT-qPCR reaction was carried out in 10 µL for each sample, including 5 µL of SYBR Green Master Mix (Roche), 1 µL of cDNA template (1:25 template dilution) and 0.7 pmol/µL of each primer. The procedure used to obtain the RT-qPCR thermal profile was: 95 °C for 20 s, 40 cycles of 95 °C for 1 s and 60 °C for 20 s. The melting curve of each amplicon was revealed by the program from 60 to 95 °C, reading every 0.5 °C. The gene-specific amplification and the absence of primer-dimers were confirmed by the presence of single peaks for all genes. qPCR was carried out in triplicate (technical replicates) on cDNA, deriving from three independent cultures (biological replicates) and each assay included three no template negative controls for each primer pair.

4.5. Nitric Oxide (NO) Determination

NO levels were measured by monitoring the formation of nitrite, the oxidation product of NO, through the Griess assay [75]. At different times from dawn, diatom samples (50 mL) were collected by centrifugation at 2600 rcf for 15 min at 4 °C (Eppendorf 5810 R, Eppendorf AG, Hamburg, Germany). The pellets were washed in phosphate buffer (KH_2PO_4 50 mM pH 7.5, 0.5 M NaCl) and centrifuged again under the same conditions. The final pellets were weighed, frozen in liquid nitrogen and kept at

−80 °C until use. Samples were homogenized in 1 mL of phosphate buffer, sonicated two times at 30% amplitude for 1 min with a one-minute-break between the two sonication cycles. The samples were centrifuged at 13,000 rcf for 15 min at 4 °C and the supernatants were analyzed for nitrite content. Aliquots (300 µL) were incubated at room temperature (25 °C) with nitrate reductase (1 U/mL) and the enzyme cofactors: flavin adenine dinucleotide (100 µM) and nicotinamide adenine dinucleotide phosphate hydrogen (0.6 mM). After 2 h, samples were treated for 10 min in the dark with 300 µL of 1% (w/v) sulphanilamide in 5% H_3PO_4 and then with 300 µL of 0.1% (w/v) N-(1-naphthy)-ethylenediamine dihydrochloride for additional 10 min. The absorbance at 540 nm was measured in 1 mL glass cuvettes and the molar concentration of nitrite in the sample was calculated by interpolation from a standard curve generated using known concentrations of sodium nitrite (0–5 µM). Nitrite content in each sample was determined in triplicate (technical replicates) on samples deriving from three independent cultures (biological replicates).

4.6. Reactive Oxygen Species (ROS) Determination

ROS levels were measured in vivo using a fluorescent ROS-sensitive dye, 2′,7′-dichlorofluorescein diacetate (H_2DCF-DA; Sigma-Aldrich, Saint Louis, MO, USA). At different times from dawn, diatom samples (15 mL) were incubated for 30 min in the dark with H_2DCF-DA (20 µM final concentration). The cells were then collected by centrifugation, as described above, homogenized in phosphate buffer (0.5 mL), and sonicated as described above. The samples were centrifuged at 13,000 rcf for 15 min at 4 °C and the supernatants were analyzed for ROS content. Aliquots (5 µL) of samples were diluted in 100 µL of MilliQ water in a 96 multiwell plate and the fluorescence was measured using excitation and emission wavelengths of 485 and 530 nm, respectively. The molar concentration of ROS in the sample was calculated from a standard curve generated using known concentrations of 2′,7′-dichlorofluorescein (H_2DCF; 0–1 µM). ROS content in each sample was determined in triplicate (technical replicates) on samples deriving from three independent cultures (biological replicates).

4.7. Thiols Determination

Three independent *S. marinoi* cultures were carried out under control (Sin150) and high sinusoidal light (Sin600) conditions. Cultures were collected at 6 h from dawn in both light conditions (i.e., at the maximal peak of light intensity) by centrifugation at 2600 rcf speed, 4 °C for 15 min (Eppendorf 5810 R, Eppendorf AG, Hamburg, Germany). Pellets were lyophilized using an Edwards lyophilizer and the dried pellets were weighed and kept at room temperature until analysis. Samples were finally analyzed by HPLC/LC–MS for ovothiol and glutathione determination, according to the protocol fully described in Milito et al., 2020 [23]. Briefly, thiols were extracted using a solution of acetonitrile:perchloric acid (1:1), reduced by adding DTT, and finally derivatized with 4-bromomethyl-7-methoxycoumarin (BMC). Samples were analyzed by reversed phase HPLC and thiol-BMC conjugates were detected with a diode-array detector at 330 nm. Isolated ovothiol-BMC adducts were characterized by High-resolution electrospray ionization mass spectrometry (HR-ESI-MS). Ovothiol B identification was confirmed by coelution with an authentic standard [23].

4.8. Data Analysis

Gene expression levels were normalized using the most stable reference genes in RT-qPCR using the sampling time 0 h (predawn) as the control condition for each experiment. Data were presented as mean ± standard error and statistical analyses were performed using the pairwise fixed reallocation randomization test by REST ($n = 3$ biological triplicate, n randomizations = 2000, relative expression software tool) [76]. Relative expression ratios above 2-fold and with p value ≤ 0.05 were considered significant. NO and ROS data were presented as mean ± standard deviation and analyzed by Kruskal–Wallis with a Dunn's post hoc test ($n = 3$ biological triplicate). Kruskal–Wallis/Dunn's test and linear correlation analyses (Pearson) were performed using PAST software package, version 3.14 [77]. Graphs were built using GraphPad Prism software V 6.01.

4.9. Nitric Oxide Synthase (Nos) Protein Sequence Analysis

The three *Homo sapiens* Nos protein sequences were downloaded from the NCBI protein database (iNOS-inducible: NP_000616.3, eNOS-endothelial: BAA05652.1 and nNOS-neuronal: NP_000611.1). The two *S. marinoi* (strain CCMP2092) Nos protein sequences were previously identified in *S. marinoi* [40], and were downloaded from the MMETSP website (Nos1 ID: MMETSP1039-20121108|3976_1; Nos2 ID: MMETSP1039-20121108|3419_1). The sequences were aligned using ClustalX and edited with GeneDoc software. The analysis of domains was performed using InterPro database.

Supplementary Materials: The following are available online at http://www.mdpi.com/1660-3397/18/9/477/s1, Figure S1: Protein sequence alignment of *S. marinoi* Nos's with human isoforms, Figure S2: *S. marinoi* growth curves, Table S1: *S. marinoi* cell growth rates and Table S2: Genes analyzed by RT-qPCR.

Author Contributions: Conceptualization, A.M., I.C., C.B., A.P.; formal analysis, A.M.; funding acquisition, A.P.; investigation, A.M., I.O., A.S.; project administration, C.B., A.P.; resources, C.B., A.P.; supervision, I.C., A.N., C.B., A.P.; validation, A.M., I.O., A.S., I.C., A.N., C.B., A.P.; visualization, A.M.; writing—original draft preparation, A.M.; writing—review and editing, A.M., I.O., A.S., I.C., A.N., C.B., A.P.; All authors have read and agreed to the published version of the manuscript.

Funding: This research received no external funding. A.M. and A.S. were supported by SZN Ph.D fellowships via the Open University.

Acknowledgments: We are grateful to Federico Corato from the Department of Research Infrastructures for Marine Biological Resources, SZN, for the set-up of the LED illumination system. We thank Florian P. Seebeck from the Department of Chemistry, University of Basel, for thiols determination analyses and for helpful discussion on an early draft of this work.

Conflicts of Interest: The authors declare no conflict of interest.

References

1. Nelson, D.M.; Treguer, P.; Brzezinski, M.A.; Leynaert, A.; Queguiner, B. Production and dissolution of biogenic silica in the ocean: Revised global estimates, comparison with regional data and relationship to biogenic sedimentation. *Global Biogeochem. Cycles* **1995**, *9*, 359–372. [CrossRef]
2. Falkowski, P.G.; Raven, J.A. *Aquatic Photosynthesis*, 2nd ed.; Princeton University Press: Princeton, NJ, USA, 2007.
3. Barra, L.; Chandrasekaran, R.; Corato, F.; Brunet, C. The Challenge of Ecophysiological Biodiversity for Biotechnological Applications of Marine Microalgae. *Mar. Drugs* **2014**, *12*, 1641–1675. [CrossRef] [PubMed]
4. Li, H.Y.; Lu, Y.; Zheng, J.W.; Yang, W.D.; Liu, J.S. Biochemical and genetic engineering of diatoms for polyunsaturated fatty acid biosynthesis. *Mar. Drugs* **2014**, *12*, 153–166. [CrossRef] [PubMed]
5. Dolch, L.J.; Marechal, E. Inventory of fatty acid desaturases in the pennate diatom *Phaeodactylum tricornutum*. *Mar. Drugs* **2015**, *13*, 1317–1339. [CrossRef]
6. Baldisserotto, C.; Sabia, A.; Ferroni, L.; Pancaldi, S. Biological aspects and biotechnological potential of marine diatoms in relation to different light regimens. *World J. Microbiol. Biotechnol.* **2019**, *35*, 35. [CrossRef]
7. Galasso, C.; Gentile, A.; Orefice, I.; Ianora, A.; Bruno, A.; Noonan, D.M.; Sansone, C.; Albini, A.; Brunet, C. Microalgal Derivatives as Potential Nutraceutical and Food Supplements for Human Health: A Focus on Cancer Prevention and Interception. *Nutrients* **2019**, *11*, 1226. [CrossRef]
8. Montsant, A.; Allen, A.E.; Coesel, S.; Martino, A.D.; Falciatore, A.; Mangogna, M.; Siaut, M.; Heijde, M.; Jabbari, K.; Maheswari, U.; et al. Identification and comparative genomic analysis of signaling and regulatory components in the diatom *Thalassiosira pseudonana*. *J. Phycol.* **2007**, *43*, 585–604. [CrossRef]
9. Parker, M.S.; Mock, T.; Armbrust, E.V. Genomic Insights into Marine Microalgae. *Annu. Rev. Genet.* **2008**, *42*, 619–645. [CrossRef]
10. Kooistra, W.H.; Gersonde, R.; Medlin, L.K.; Mann, D.G. The Origin and Evolution of the Diatoms: Their Adaptation to a Planktonic Existence. In *Evolution of Primary Producers in the Sea*; Falkowski, P.G., Knoll, A.H., Eds.; Academic Press: Burlington, MA, USA, 2007; pp. 207–249.
11. Vardi, A. Cell signaling in marine diatoms. *Commun. Integr. Biol.* **2008**, *1*, 134–136. [CrossRef]
12. Bowler, C.; Allen, A.E.; Badger, J.H.; Grimwood, J.; Jabbari, K.; Kuo, A.; Maheswari, U.; Martens, C.; Maumus, F.; Otillar, R.P.; et al. The *Phaeodactylum* genome reveals the evolutionary history of diatom genomes. *Nature* **2008**, *456*, 239–244. [CrossRef]

13. Armbrust, E.V. The life of diatoms in the world's oceans. *Nature* **2009**, *459*, 185–192. [CrossRef] [PubMed]
14. Brunet, C.; Chandrasekaran, R.; Barra, L.; Giovagnetti, V.; Corato, F.; Ruban, A.V. Spectral radiation dependent photoprotective mechanism in the diatom *Pseudo-nitzschia multistriata*. *PLoS ONE* **2004**, *9*, e87015. [CrossRef] [PubMed]
15. Bertrand, M. Carotenoid biosynthesis in diatoms. *Photosynth. Res.* **2010**, *106*, 89–102. [CrossRef] [PubMed]
16. Chandrasekaran, R.; Barra, L.; Carillo, S.; Caruso, T.; Corsaro, M.M.; Dal Piaz, F.; Graziani, G.; Corato, F.; Pepe, D.; Manfredonia, A.; et al. Light modulation of biomass and macromolecular composition of the diatom *Skeletonema marinoi*. *J. Biotechnol.* **2014**, *192*, 114–122. [CrossRef]
17. Orefice, I.; Chandrasekaran, R.; Smerilli, A.; Corato, F.; Caruso, T.; Casillo, A.; Corsaro, M.M.; Dal Piaz, F.; Ruban, A.V.; Brunet, C. Light-induced changes in the photosynthetic physiology and biochemistry in the diatom *Skeletonema marinoi*. *Algal Res.* **2016**, *17*, 1–13. [CrossRef]
18. Smerilli, A.; Orefice, I.; Corato, F.; Gavalas Olea, A.; Ruban, A.V.; Brunet, C. Photoprotective and antioxidant responses to light spectrum and intensity variations in the coastal diatom *Skeletonema marinoi*. *Environ. Microbiol.* **2017**, *19*, 611–627. [CrossRef]
19. Smerilli, A.; Balzano, S.; Maselli, M.; Blasio, M.; Orefice, I.; Galasso, C.; Sansone, C.; Brunet, C. Antioxidant and Photoprotection Networking in the Coastal Diatom *Skeletonema marinoi*. *Antioxidants* **2019**, *8*, 154. [CrossRef]
20. Kirk, J.T.O. Thermal dissociation of fucoxanthin-protein binding in pigment complexes from chloroplasts of *Hormosira* (phaeophyta). *Plant Sci. Lett.* **1977**, *9*, 373–380. [CrossRef]
21. Müller, P.; Li, X.-P.; Niyogi, K.K. Non-Photochemical Quenching. A Response to Excess Light Energy. *Plant Physiol.* **2001**, *125*, 1558–1566. [CrossRef]
22. Lavaud, J. Fast Regulation of Photosynthesis in Diatoms: Mechanisms, Evolution and Ecophysiology. *Funct. Plant Sci. Biotechnol.* **2007**, *1*, 267–287.
23. Milito, A.; Castellano, I.; Burn, R.; Seebeck, F.P.; Brunet, C.; Palumbo, A. First evidence of ovothiol biosynthesis in marine diatoms. *Free Radic. Biol. Med.* **2020**, *152*, 680–688. [CrossRef] [PubMed]
24. Turner, E.; Klevit, R.; Hager, L.J.; Shapiro, B.M. Ovothiols, a family of redox-active mercaptohistidine compounds from marine invertebrate eggs. *Biochemistry* **1987**, *26*, 4028–4036. [CrossRef] [PubMed]
25. Palumbo, A.; Castellano, I.; Napolitano, A. Ovothiol: A potent natural antioxidant from marine organisms. In *Blue Biotechnology. Production and Use of Marine Molecules. Part 2: Marine Molecules for Disease Treatment/Prevention and for Biological Research*; La Barre, S., Bates, S.S., Eds.; Wiley VCH: Weinheim, DE, USA, 2018; pp. 583–610.
26. Weaver, K.H.; Rabenstein, D.L. Thiol/Disulfide Exchange Reactions of Ovothiol A with Glutathione. *J. Org. Chem.* **1995**, *60*, 1904–1907. [CrossRef]
27. Marjanovic, B.; Simic, M.G.; Jovanovic, S.V. Heterocyclic thiols as antioxidants: Why Ovothiol C is a better antioxidant than ergothioneine. *Free Radic. Biol. Med.* **1995**, *18*, 679–685. [CrossRef]
28. Ariyanayagam, M.R.; Fairlamb, A.H. Ovothiol and trypanothione as antioxidants in trypanosomatids. *Mol. Biochem. Parasitol.* **2001**, *115*, 189–198. [CrossRef]
29. Jacob, C. A scent of therapy: Pharmacological implications of natural products containing redox-active sulfur atoms. *Nat. Prod. Rep.* **2006**, *23*, 851–863. [CrossRef]
30. Brancaccio, M.; D'Argenio, G.; Lembo, V.; Palumbo, A.; Castellano, I. Antifibrotic Effect of Marine Ovothiol in an In Vivo Model of Liver Fibrosis. *Oxid. Med. Cell Longev.* **2018**, *2018*, 5045734. [CrossRef]
31. Milito, A.; Brancaccio, M.; D'Argenio, G.; Castellano, I. Natural Sulfur-Containing Compounds: An Alternative Therapeutic Strategy against Liver Fibrosis. *Cells* **2019**, *8*, 1356. [CrossRef]
32. Russo, G.L.; Russo, M.; Castellano, I.; Napolitano, A.; Palumbo, A. Ovothiol isolated from sea urchin oocytes induces autophagy in the Hep-G2 cell line. *Mar. Drugs* **2014**, *12*, 4069–4085. [CrossRef]
33. Brancaccio, M.; Russo, M.; Masullo, M.; Palumbo, A.; Russo, G.L.; Castellano, I. Sulfur-containing histidine compounds inhibit γ-glutamyl transpeptidase activity in human cancer cells. *J. Biol. Chem.* **2019**, *294*, 14603–14614. [CrossRef]
34. Milito, A.; Brancaccio, M.; Lisurek, M.; Masullo, M.; Palumbo, A.; Castellano, I. Probing the Interactions of Sulfur-Containing Histidine Compounds with Human Gamma-Glutamyl Transpeptidase. *Mar. Drugs* **2019**, *17*, 650. [CrossRef] [PubMed]

35. Castellano, I.; Di Tomo, P.; Di Pietro, N.; Mandatori, D.; Pipino, C.; Formoso, G.; Napolitano, A.; Palumbo, A. Anti-Inflammatory Activity of Marine Ovothiol A in an In Vitro Model of Endothelial Dysfunction Induced by Hyperglycemia. *Oxid. Med. Cell. Longev.* **2018**, *2018*, 2087373. [CrossRef] [PubMed]
36. Braunshausen, A.; Seebeck, F.P. Identification and Characterization of the First Ovothiol Biosynthetic Enzyme. *J. Am. Chem. Soc.* **2011**, *133*, 1757–1759. [CrossRef] [PubMed]
37. Naowarojna, N.; Huang, P.; Cai, Y.; Song, H.; Wu, L.; Cheng, R.; Li, Y.; Wang, S.; Lyu, H.; Zhang, L.; et al. In Vitro Reconstitution of the Remaining Steps in Ovothiol A Biosynthesis: C–S Lyase and Methyltransferase Reactions. *Org. Lett.* **2018**, *20*, 5427–5430. [CrossRef]
38. Selman-Reimer, S.; Duhe, R.J.; Stockman, B.J.; Selman, B.R. L-1-N-methyl-4-mercaptohistidine disulfide, a potential endogenous regulator in the redox control of chloroplast coupling factor 1 in *Dunaliella*. *J. Biol. Chem.* **1991**, *266*, 182–188.
39. O'Neill, E.C.; Trick, M.; Hill, L.; Rejzek, M.; Dusi, R.G.; Hamilton, C.J.; Zimba, P.V.; Henrissat, B.; Field, R.A. The transcriptome of *Euglena gracilis* reveals unexpected metabolic capabilities for carbohydrate and natural product biochemistry. *Mol. Biosyst.* **2015**, *11*, 2808–2820. [CrossRef]
40. Crawford, N.M.; Guo, F.-Q. New insights into nitric oxide metabolism and regulatory functions. *Trends Plant Sci.* **2005**, *10*, 195–200. [CrossRef]
41. Gechev, T.S.; Van Breusegem, F.; Stone, J.M.; Denev, I.; Laloi, C. Reactive oxygen species as signals that modulate plant stress responses and programmed cell death. *BioEssays* **2006**, *28*, 1091–1101. [CrossRef]
42. Grün, S.; Lindermayr, C.; Sell, S.; Durner, J. Nitric oxide and gene regulation in plants. *J. Exp. Bot.* **2006**, *57*, 507–516. [CrossRef]
43. Gallina, A.A.; Brunet, C.; Palumbo, A.; Casotti, R. The Effect of Polyunsaturated Aldehydes on *Skeletonema marinoi* (Bacillariophyceae): The Involvement of Reactive Oxygen Species and Nitric Oxide. *Mar. Drugs* **2014**, *12*, 4165–4187. [CrossRef]
44. Di Dato, V.; Musacchia, F.; Petrosino, G.; Patil, S.; Montresor, M.; Sanges, R.; Ferrante, M.I. Transcriptome sequencing of three *Pseudo-nitzschia* species reveals comparable gene sets and the presence of *Nitric Oxide Synthase* genes in diatoms. *Sci. Rep.* **2015**, *5*, 12329. [CrossRef] [PubMed]
45. Barra, L.; Ruggiero, M.V.; Sarno, D.; Montresor, M.; Kooistra, W.H.C.F. Strengths and weaknesses of microarray approaches to detect *Pseudo-nitzschia* species in the field. *Environ. Sci. Pollut. Res. Int.* **2013**, *20*, 6705–6718. [CrossRef] [PubMed]
46. Andreakis, N.; D'Aniello, S.; Albalat, R.; Patti, F.P.; Garcia-Fernàndez, J.; Procaccini, G.; Sordino, P.; Palumbo, A. Evolution of the Nitric Oxide Synthase Family in Metazoans. *Mol. Biol. Evol.* **2011**, *28*, 163–179. [CrossRef] [PubMed]
47. Shapiro, B.M. The control of oxidant stress at fertilization. *Science* **1991**, *252*, 533–536. [CrossRef]
48. Castellano, I.; Migliaccio, O.; D'Aniello, S.; Merlino, A.; Napolitano, A.; Palumbo, A. Shedding light on ovothiol biosynthesis in marine metazoans. *Sci. Rep.* **2016**, *6*, 21506. [CrossRef]
49. Yanshole, V.V.; Yanshole, L.V.; Zelentsova, E.A.; Tsentalovich, Y.P. Ovothiol A is the Main Antioxidant in Fish Lens. *Metabolites* **2019**, *9*, 95. [CrossRef]
50. Spies, H.S.; Steenkamp, D.J. Thiols of intracellular pathogens. Identification of ovothiol A in *Leishmania donovani* and structural analysis of a novel thiol from *Mycobacterium bovis*. *Europ. J. Biochem.* **1994**, *224*, 203–213. [CrossRef]
51. Tarrant, A.M.; Payton, S.L.; Reitzel, A.M.; Porter, D.T.; Jenny, M.J. Ultraviolet radiation significantly enhances the molecular response to dispersant and sweet crude oil exposure in *Nematostella vectensis*. *Mar. Environ. Res.* **2018**, *134*, 96–108. [CrossRef]
52. Diaz de Cerio, O.; Reina, L.; Squatrito, V.; Etxebarria, N.; Gonzalez-Gaya, B.; Cancio, I. Gametogenesis-Related Fluctuations in Ovothiol Levels in the Mantle of Mussels from Different Estuaries: Fighting Oxidative Stress for Spawning in Polluted Waters. *Biomolecules* **2020**, *10*, 373. [CrossRef]
53. Rohl, I.; Schneider, B.; Schmidt, B.; Zeeck, E. L-ovothiol A: The egg release pheromone of the marine polychaete *Platynereis Dumerilii*: Anellida: Polychaeta. *Z. Naturforsch. C J. Biosci.* **1999**, *54*, 1145–1147. [CrossRef]
54. Castellano, I.; Seebeck, F.P. On ovothiol biosynthesis and biological roles: From life in the ocean to therapeutic potential. *Nat. Prod. Rep.* **2018**, *35*, 1241–1250. [CrossRef] [PubMed]

55. Gerdol, M.; Sollitto, M.; Pallavicini, A.; Castellano, I. The complex evolutionary history of sulfoxide synthase in ovothiol biosynthesis. *Proc. R. Soc. B* **2019**, *286*, 20191812. [CrossRef] [PubMed]
56. Kennedy, F.; Martin, A.; McMinn, A. Insights into the Production and Role of Nitric Oxide in the Antarctic Sea-ice Diatom Fragilariopsis cylindrus. *J. Phycol.* **2020**, in press. [CrossRef] [PubMed]
57. Sassenhagen, I.; Wilken, S.; Godhe, A.; Rengefors, K. Phenotypic plasticity and differentiation in an invasive freshwater microalga. *Harmful Algae* **2015**, *41*, 38–45. [CrossRef]
58. Chung, T.-Y.; Kuo, C.-Y.; Lin, W.-J.; Wang, W.-L.; Chou, J.-Y. Indole-3-acetic-acid-induced phenotypic plasticity in *Desmodesmus* algae. *Sci Rep* **2018**, *8*, 10270. [CrossRef]
59. Lin, W.-J.; Ho, H.-C.; Chu, S.-C.; Chou, J.-Y. Effects of auxin derivatives on phenotypic plasticity and stress tolerance in five species of the green alga *Desmodesmus* (Chlorophyceae, Chlorophyta). *Peer J.* **2020**, *8*, e8623. [CrossRef]
60. Giovagnetti, V.; Flori, S.; Tramontano, F.; Lavaud, J.; Brunet, C. The Velocity of Light Intensity Increase Modulates the Photoprotective Response in Coastal Diatoms. *PLoS ONE* **2014**, *9*, e103782. [CrossRef]
61. Fu, W.; Nelson, D.; Yi, Z.; Xu, M.; Khraiwesh, B.; Jijakli, K.; Chaiboonchoe, A.; Alzahmi, A.; Al-Khairy, D.; Brynjolfsson, S.; et al. Bioactive Compounds From Microalgae: Current Development and Prospects. In *Studies in Natural Products Chemistry*; Rahman, A., Ed.; Elsevier: Amsterdam, The Netherlands, 2017; pp. 199–225.
62. Sansone, C.; Brunet, C. Promises and Challenges of Microalgal Antioxidant Production. *Antioxidants* **2019**, *8*, 199. [CrossRef]
63. Orefice, I.; Musella, M.; Smerilli, A.; Sansone, C.; Chandrasekaran, R.; Corato, F.; Brunet, C. Role of nutrient concentrations and water movement on diatom's productivity in culture. *Sci. Rep.* **2019**, *9*, 1479. [CrossRef]
64. Kourtchenko, O.; Rajala, T.; Godhe, A. Growth of a common planktonic diatom quantified using solid medium culturing. *Sci. Rep.* **2018**, *8*, 9757. [CrossRef]
65. Liao, I.C.; Su, H.M.; Lin, J.H. Larval foods for Penaeid prawns. In *CRC Handbook of Mariculture, Volume I: Crustacean Aquaculture*; McVey, J.P., Ed.; CRC Press: Boca Raton, FL, USA, 1993; pp. 29–59.
66. Su, H.M.; Lei, C.H.; Liao, I.C. Effect of temperature, illumination and salinity on the growth rates of *Skeletonema costatum. J. Fish Soc. Taiwan* **1990**, *17*, 213–222.
67. Coutteau, P.; Sorgeloos, P. The use of algal substitutes and the requirement for live algae in the hatchery and nursery rearing of bivalve molluscs: An international survey. *J. Shellfish Res.* **1992**, *11*, 467–476.
68. Brown, M.R.; Jeffrey, S.W.; Volkman, J.K.; Dunstan, G.A. Nutritional properties of microalgae for mariculture. *Aquaculture* **1997**, *151*, 315–331. [CrossRef]
69. Miralto, A.; Barone, G.; Romano, G.; Poulet, S.A.; Ianora, A.; Russo, G.L.; Buttino, I.; Mazzarella, G.; Laabir, M.; Cabrini, M.; et al. The insidious effect of diatoms on copepod reproduction. *Nature* **1999**, *402*, 173–176. [CrossRef]
70. Guillard, R.R.L. Culture of Phytoplankton for Feeding Marine Invertebrates. In *Culture of Marine Invertebrate Animals*; Smith, W.L., Chanley, M.H., Eds.; Springer: Boston, MA, USA, 1975; pp. 29–60.
71. Brunet, C.; Johnsen, G.; Lavaud, J.; Roy, S. Pigments and photoacclimation processes. In *Phytoplankton Pigments: Characterization, Chemotaxonomy and Applications in Oceanography*; Roy, S., Llewellyn, C.A., Egeland, E.S., Johnsen, G., Eds.; Cambridge University Press: Cambridge, UK, 2011; pp. 445–471.
72. Orefice, I.; Lauritano, C.; Procaccini, G.; Ianora, A.; Romano, G. Insights into possible cell-death markers in the diatom *Skeletonema marinoi* in response to senescence and silica starvation. *Mar. Genomics* **2015**, *24*, 81–88. [CrossRef]
73. Pfaffl, M.W.; Tichopad, A.; Prgomet, C.; Neuvians, T.P. Determination of stable housekeeping genes, differentially regulated target genes and sample integrity: BestKeeper—Excel-based tool using pair-wise correlations. *Biotechnol. Lett.* **2004**, *26*, 509–515. [CrossRef]
74. Andersen, C.L.; Jensen, J.L.; Ørntoft, T.F. Normalization of Real-Time Quantitative Reverse Transcription-PCR Data: A Model-Based Variance Estimation Approach to Identify Genes Suited for Normalization, Applied to Bladder and Colon Cancer Data Sets. *Cancer Res.* **2004**, *64*, 5245–5250. [CrossRef]
75. Green, L.C.; Wagner, D.A.; Glogowski, J.; Skipper, P.L.; Wishnok, J.S.; Tannenbaum, S.R. Analysis of nitrate, nitrite, and [^{15}N] nitrate in biological fluids. *Anal. Biochem.* **1982**, *126*, 131–138. [CrossRef]

76. Pfaffl, M.W.; Horgan, G.W.; Dempfle, L. Relative expression software tool (REST©) for group-wise comparison and statistical analysis of relative expression results in real-time PCR. *Nucleic Acids Res.* **2002**, *30*, e36. [CrossRef]
77. Hammer, Ø.; Harper, D.A.T.; Ryan, P.D. PAST: Paleontological Statistics Software Package for Education and Data Analysis. *Palaeontol. Electron.* **2001**, *4*, 1–9.

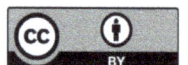

© 2020 by the authors. Licensee MDPI, Basel, Switzerland. This article is an open access article distributed under the terms and conditions of the Creative Commons Attribution (CC BY) license (http://creativecommons.org/licenses/by/4.0/).

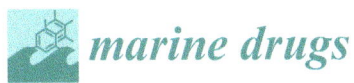

Article

Preparation, Supramolecular Aggregation and Immunological Activity of the Bona Fide Vaccine Adjuvant Sulfavant S

Emiliano Manzo [1,*,†], **Laura Fioretto** [1,2,†], **Carmela Gallo** [1], **Marcello Ziaco** [3], **Genoveffa Nuzzo** [1], **Giuliana D'Ippolito** [1], **Assunta Borzacchiello** [4], **Antonio Fabozzi** [4], **Raffaele De Palma** [1,5] and **Angelo Fontana** [1,*]

1. Bio-Organic Chemistry Unit, CNR-Institute of Biomolecular Chemistry, Via Campi Flegrei 34, 80078 Pozzuoli, Italy; l.fioretto@icb.cnr.it (L.F.); carmen.gallo@icb.cnr.it (C.G.); nuzzo.genoveffa@icb.cnr.it (G.N.); gdippolito@icb.cnr.it (G.D.); raffaele.depalma@unige.it (R.D.P.)
2. Consorzio Italbiotec, Via Fantoli, 16/15, 20138 Milano, Italy
3. BioSearch Srl., Villa Comunale c/o Stazione Zoologica "A.Dohrn", 80121 Napoli, Italy; m.ziaco@icb.cnr.it
4. Institute for Polymers, Composites and Biomaterials (IPCB), CNR, 80125 Naples, Italy; bassunta@unina.it (A.B.); Sirfabozzi@hotmail.it (A.F.)
5. Medicina Interna, Immunologia Clinica e Medicina Traslazionale, Università di Genova and IRCCS-Ospedale S. Martino, 16131 Genova, Italy
* Correspondence: emanzo@icb.cnr.it (E.M.); afontana@icb.cnr.it (A.F.)
† These authors contributed equally.

Received: 20 July 2020; Accepted: 26 August 2020; Published: 29 August 2020

Abstract: In aqueous conditions, amphiphilic bioactive molecules are able to form self-assembled colloidal structures modifying their biological activity. This behavior is generally neglected in preclinical studies, despite its impact on pharmacological development. In this regard, a significative example is represented by a new class of amphiphilic marine-inspired vaccine adjuvants, collectively named Sulfavants, based on the β-sulfoquinovosyl-diacylglyceride skeleton. The family includes the lead product Sulfavant A (**1**) and two epimers, Sulfavant R (**2**) and Sulfavant S (**3**), differing only for the stereochemistry at C-2 of glycerol. The three compounds showed a significant difference in immunological potency, presumably correlated with change of the aggregates in water. Here, a new synthesis of diastereopure **3** was achieved, and the study of the immunomodulatory behavior of mixtures of **2/3** proved that the bizarre in vitro response to **1**–**3** effectively depends on the supramolecular aggregation states, likely affecting the bioavailability of agonists that can effectively interact with the cellular targets. The evidence obtained with the mixture of pure Sulfavant R (**2**) and Sulfavant S (**3**) proves, for the first time, that supramolecular organization of a mixture of active epimers in aqueous solution can bias evaluation of their biological and pharmacological potential.

Keywords: sulfavants; adjuvant; immunomodulatory activity; colloid; aggregates

1. Introduction

Development of new drugs is a long and expensive process, and often many unpredictable problems arise in clinical phases due to the chemical-physical behavior of some molecules in physiological environments. Several pharmacologically active compounds and commercial drugs are in fact amphiphilic substances able to self-aggregate in aqueous solutions. Self-assembly in water is a spontaneous process involving the arrangement in supramolecular structures that are stabilized by non-covalent interactions and minimizes the direct contact between the hydrophobic part of the molecule and the polar solvent [1]. This behavior is as common as it is poorly considered, even if it can seriously affect biological activity and pharmacological developments. Only recently, studies have focused on the relevance of physicochemical properties, such as lipophilicity, in the in vitro selection of drug candidates and likelihood of success in development [2]. In fact, molecular aggregation can be critical in determining in vivo ADMET (absorption, distribution, metabolism, excretion, and toxicity) properties, but also in affecting the overall quality of a drug candidate in cellular assays. In physiological media, lipophilic substances produce complex equilibria involving free molecules and many aggregates differing in size and shape. Therefore, as aggregates are not involved in the pharmacodynamic interaction, these equilibria determine the effective concentration of the bioactive product on the target and in cellular tests.

Adjuvants are chemical components that are combined with antigens to enhance the immune response to vaccines [3]. Traditionally, adjuvants are composed of a suspension of insoluble compounds (e.g., oils, aluminum, particulate materials containing small molecules) in water. In the last few years, a major breakthrough has been the discovery of the link between adjuvants and innate immune response triggered by antigen-presenting cells (APCs) that capture and process antigens for presentation to T-lymphocytes, and to produce signals required for the proliferation and differentiation of lymphocytes [4–11]. In particular, the identification of pattern recognition receptors (PRRs) as primary effectors of the plastic activation of APCs has rapidly led to the rational design of molecular adjuvants based on single, immunomodulatory molecules. In this context, we recently characterized β-sulfoquinovosyl-diacyl glycerols (β-SQDGs) as a novel class of vaccine adjuvants collectively named Sulfavants. These synthetic molecules were inspired by natural and marine α-sulfoquinovosyl-diacylglycerols (α-SQDGs) occurring as membrane constituents in photosynthetic organisms [12–15]. Sulfavant A (**1**) (1,2-O-distearoyl-3-O-(β-sulfoquinovosyl)-*R/S*-glycerol), the prototype of the family, induces maturation of human dendritic cells (hDCs) at micromolar concentrations with a typical "bell-shaped" dose–response curve that is featured by a maximum around 10 µM. Sulfavant A (**1**) also showed promising adjuvant activity in *in vivo* experiments, as it was able both to boost immune protection in mice and to inhibit tumor growth in an experimental model of cancer vaccine against melanoma [13–15].

Sulfavant A (**1**)

Compound **1** is a 1.3:1 mixture of *R/S* epimers at carbon 2 of glycerol moiety. In order to investigate the pharmacological properties of this new class of molecules, we also synthetized two enantiopure analogues named Sulfavant R (**2**) and S (**3**) [12]. Surprisingly, compound **2** showed maturation of hDCs at nanomolar concentrations with 1000-fold increase of the activity in comparison to the epimeric mixture **1**. We never had the opportunity to test rigorously the biological response to pure Sulfavant S (**3**) because of a partial loss of stereospecificity of the synthesis for this product due to a fast process of opening and closure of the *S*-glycerol acetonide during the glycosylation step (Scheme 1) [12]. However, a fraction containing 80% Sulfavant S (**3**) and 20% Sulfavant R (**2**) was also active on DCs but at concentrations between those of **1** and **2**. All of these compounds gave bell-shaped concentration–response curves, and chemo-physical analysis revealed a clear correlation between size of the microparticles in water and activation of hDC maturation [12].

Sulfavant R (**2**) Sulfavant S (**3**)

In the present work, we implemented a stereospecific synthesis of Sulfavant S (3) with the aim to prove that the immunological priming of hDC by the enantiopure isomers is significantly dependent, per se, on the type of aggregation of active products.

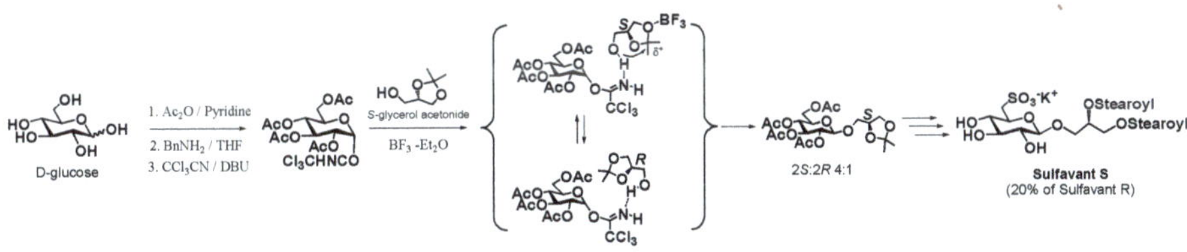

Scheme 1. Literature synthetic approach for the preparation of Sulfavant S (3) (with 20% of R epimer) according to Manzo et al., 2019 [12].

2. Results and Discussion

The use of (R)-(-)-1,2-isopropylideneglycerol as an acceptor in the coupling step with the trichloroacetamidate sugar gave high stereospecificity for the synthesis of Sulfavant R (2) [12]. However, a similar reaction with (S)-(+)-1,2-isopropylideneglycerol led to a low diastereoselective yield because of opening and closure of the acetonide ring under acidic conditions due to the boron trifluoride catalyst. As described in Scheme 1, formation of a complex between boron trifluoride and the acetonide oxygen atoms can start a fast and reversible process of racemization at C-2 of glycerol. The rearrangement rate was comparable to formation of the glycosidic bond, thus resulting in 20% epimerization of the glycosylated product. In order to overcome this issue, we prepared an alternative acceptor for the glycosylation reaction (Scheme 2).

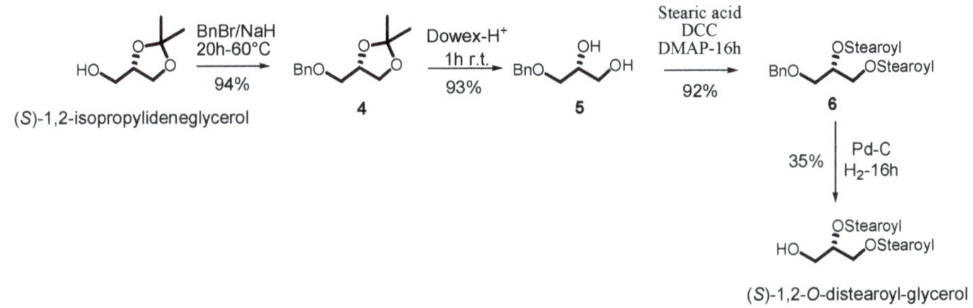

Scheme 2. Synthesis of the acceptor (S)-1,2-O-distearoylglycerol.

Starting from the usual S-1,2-isopropylideneglycerol, the first step was the protection of the primary hydroxy group by benzylation with benzyl bromide and sodium hydride. Treatment with Dowex H$^+$ led to the diol derivative (5) from which the distearoyl-benzyl intermediate (6) was obtained by acylation with stearic acid and N,N'-dicyclohexylcarbodiimide. Without affecting the chirality of the stereocenter at C-2 of glycerol, debenzylation by hydrogenolysis on palladium gave the (S)-1,2-O-distearoylglycerol acceptor with 35% overall yield. The new acceptor was immediately coupled with the peracetylated glucosyl-trichloroacetimidate donor without loss of stereospecificity. As shown in Scheme 3, after deacetylation of the sugar moiety by hydrazinolysis, the synthesis of the sulfolipid followed the same sequence of reactions previously reported to give pure Sulfavant S [12] (Figure 1).

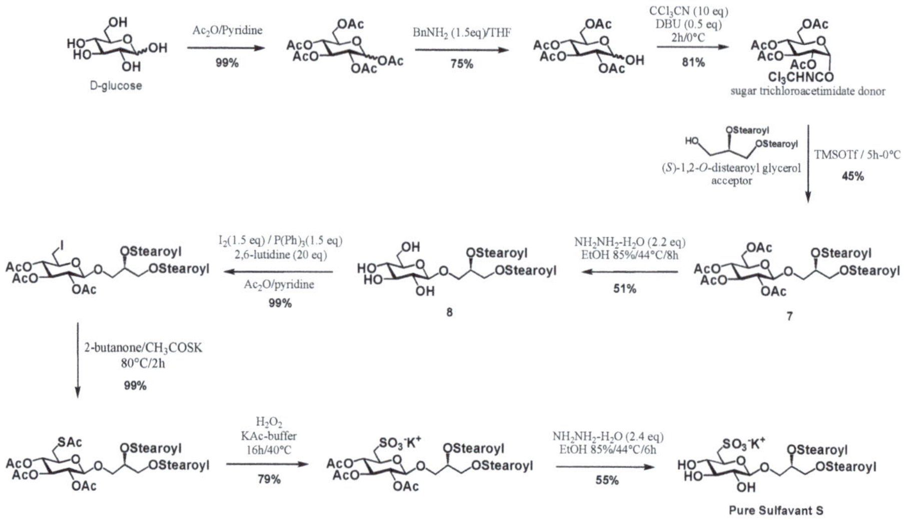

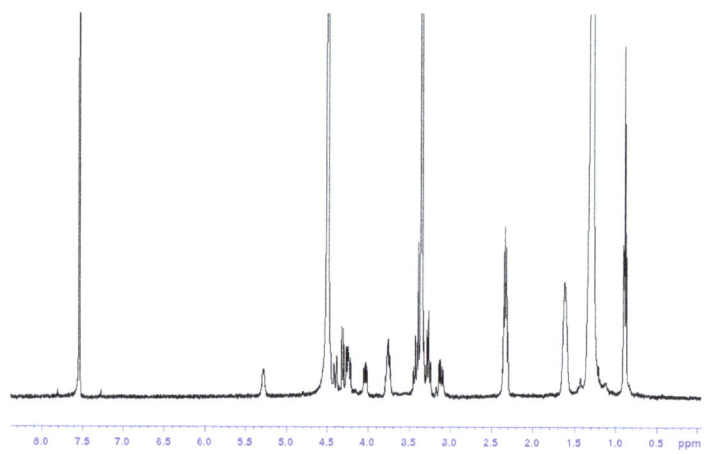

Scheme 3. Synthesis of the diastereopure Sulfavant S (**3**).

Figure 1. ^{1}H-NMR of pure **3** in CDCl$_3$:CD$_3$OD 1:1 at 600MHz.

Enantiopure Sulfavant S (**3**) was tested for the activation of hDCs derived from blood monocytes [13]. DCs are the most efficient antigen-presenting cells (APCs) [16–22], often called "nature's adjuvant" [23] for their ability to induce activation and specific expansion of CD4$^+$ helper T (Th) and CD8$^+$ cytotoxic T (CTL) lymphocytes. The search for substances able to activate and prepare DCs to face pathogens represents a key tool in the development of new molecular adjuvants for vaccines against tumors or infections [24–26]. The effect of compound **3** on hDC maturation was measured by upregulation of CD83, an integral membrane protein belonging to the immunoglobulin superfamily and selectively expressed on mature DCs [27]. The activity of pure Sulfavant S (**3**) was similar to that of Sulfavant R (**2**) [12], with maximum CD83 expression at nanomolar concentration (Figure 2).

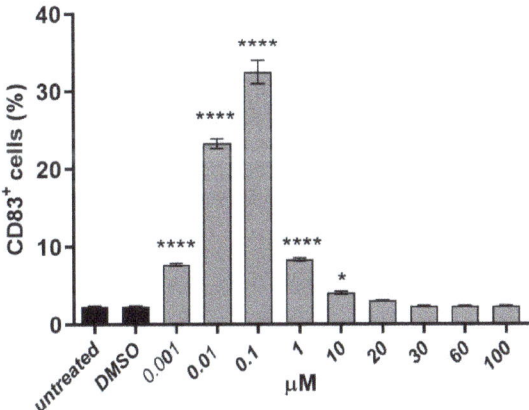

Figure 2. Percentage of CD83$^+$ cells stimulated by pure Sulfavant S (**3**); asterisks indicate significant differences from untreated cells; * $p < 0.5$, **** $p < 0.0001$.

In addition, as previously observed for compounds **1** and **2**, Sulfavant S (**3**) gave a bell-shaped dose activity curve that is common to other lipophilic drugs and reflects the formation of aggregates in the aqueous media [28–32]. In confirmation, Dynamic Light Scattering (DLS) measurements showed that pure **3** formed very small colloidal particles with a hydrodynamic radius of about 50 nm. The size of these particles was very similar to those we have previously observed for the epimer Sulfavant R (**2**) [12], thus proving that pure isomers have very similar biological and chemo-physical properties. Notably, both compounds were 1000-fold more active than Sulfavant A (**1**), which is composed of a 1.3:1 mixture of **2** and **3**.

In order to test the effect of the aggregation on the immunological response and to test our hypothesis on the reduction of the activity due to mixing of the two active epimers, we analyzed the effect of different combinations of Sulfavant R and Sulfavant S on hDC maturation.

Sulfavant R (**2**) was slightly more active than Sulfavant S (**3**), but their mixtures were always less effective in triggering CD83 expression than the pure molecules (Figure 3A). The addition of the *S* epimer (**3**) to the *R* epimer (**2**) determined a linear decrease of the activity in the range from 100% to 40% of *R*. Further additions revert the response (20% and 0% of *R*) as expected for the formation of mixture where the *S* epimer became progressively predominant. Furthermore, in complete agreement with the response elicited by **1**, the immunomodulatory activity increased to micromolar concentrations by mixture of **2** and **3** with a 1.3:1 ratio, which is identical to the composition of Sulfavant A (**1**) (Figure 3B). On the whole, these experiments proved that the mixing ratio can significantly affect the activity of amphiphilic compounds. In the case of Sulfavants, there is an incredibly large difference between potency of pure products and their mixture, thus determining erroneous evaluation of the therapeutic potential.

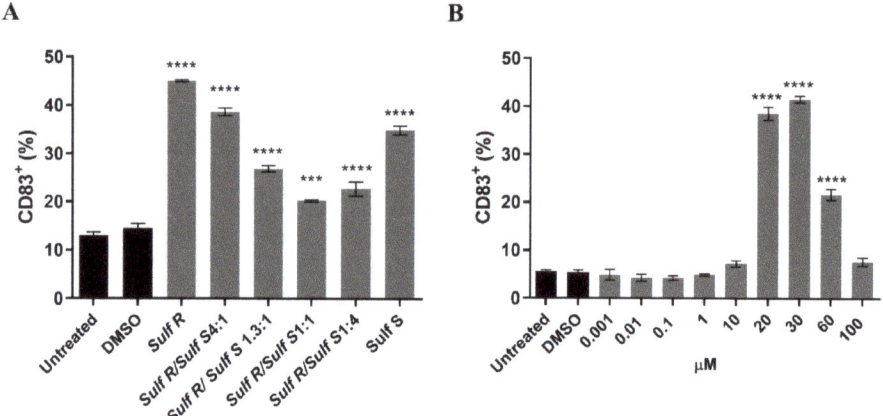

Figure 3. Effect of combination of **2** and **3** on hDC maturation. (**A**) CD83+ DC cells triggered by different combinations of **2** and **3** at an overall concentration of 0.1 µM; (**B**) CD83+ DC cells triggered by 1.3:1 mixture of **2** and **3** at concentrations from 1 nM to 100 µM; asterisks indicate significant differences from untreated cells; *** $p < 0.001$, **** $p < 0.0001$.

In order to test the role of aggregation on changes of the biological activity of **1–3**, we characterized the suspension of pure products and their mixture in water by Dynamic Light Scattering (DLS) (Figure 4).

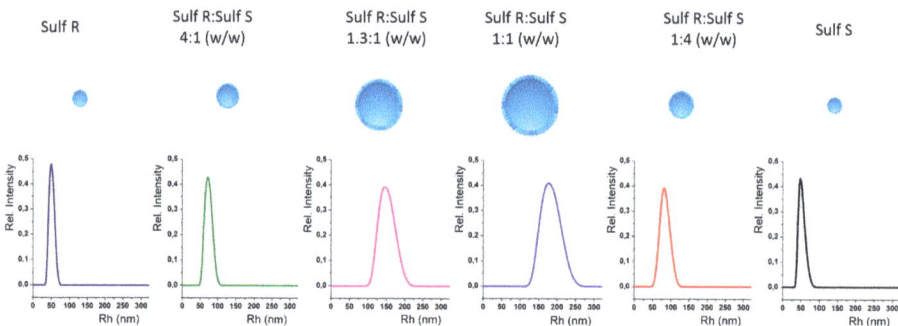

Figure 4. Effect of combination of **2** and **3** on the hydrodynamic radius evaluated by means of Dynamic Light Scattering.

DLS measures showed a constant increase of the aggregate size moving from Sulfavant R (**2**) (about 50 nm) to the 1:1 mixture of Sulfavant R (**2**) and Sulfavant S (**3**) (about 170 nm). In analogy with the effect on the biological activity, further additions of compound **3** shrank the particle up to 50 nm of the pure Sulfavant S (**3**). This surprising behavior was linked to the different way that Sulfavants self-organize in aqueous solution [12]. The evidence that almost identical bioactive molecules (like epimers) could dramatically lose the biological activity as a result of their mixing represents a new paradigm to be evaluated in the study of bioactive lipophilic substances. We have previously suggested that the stability of the final aggregates has a relevant role in influencing the effective bioavailability of free active molecules in equilibrium with self-aggregates [12]. The current results obtained with a mixture of pure Sulfavant R (**2**) and Sulfavant S (**3**) prove, for the first time, that supramolecular organization of mixture of active epimers in aqueous solutions can bias evaluation of their biological and pharmacological potential.

3. Materials and Methods

NMR spectra were recorded on a Bruker Avance-400 (400.13 MHz) and on a Bruker DRX-600 equipped with a TXI CryoProbe in CDCl$_3$ and in CDCl$_3$:CD$_3$OD 1:1 (δ values referred to CHCl$_3$ and CH$_3$OH at 7.26 and 3.34 ppm respectively). HR-MS spectra were acquired by a Q-Exactive Hybrid Quadrupole-Orbitrap mass spectrometer (Thermo Scientific, Waltham, MA, USA). TLC plates (Kieselgel 60 F$_{254}$) and silica gel powder (Kieselgel 60, 0.063–0.200 mm) were from Merck.

All the reagents were purchased from Sigma-Aldrich and used without any further purification. DLS measurements were performed with a homemade instrument composed with a Photocor compact goniometer, a SMD 6000 Laser Quantum 50 mW light source operating at 5325 Å, a photomultiplier (PMT-120-OP/B) and a correlator (Flex02-01D, Correlator.com).

3.1. Dynamic Light Scattering (DLS)

Measurements were performed at (25.00 ± 0.05) °C with temperature controlled through the use of a thermostat bath. In DLS, the intensity autocorrelation function, g$^{(2)}$(t), was measured for the instrument configuration corresponding to the scattering angle of 90°. The intensity autocorrelation function is related to the electric field autocorrelation function through the Siegert relation. The electric field autocorrelation function, g$^{(1)}$(t), is defined as

$$g^{(1)}(t) = \int_{-\infty}^{+\infty} \tau A(\tau) \exp\left(-\frac{t}{\tau}\right) d\ln \tau \quad (1)$$

where $\tau = 1/\Gamma$ and q is the modulus of the scattering vector $q = 4\lambda n_0/\lambda \sin(\theta/2)$, $n_0 = 1.33$ is the refractive index of the solvent, λ is the incident wavelength and θ represents the scattering angle. Evaluation of the relaxation rate Γ distribution allows calculating the translational diffusion coefficient: $D = \Gamma/q^2$: (J. B. a. R. Pecora, Dynamic Light Scattering: With Applications to Chemistry, Biology, and Physics, Couvire Dover Publications, 2003.)

Inverse Laplace transforms were performed using a variation of the CONTIN algorithm incorporated in Precision Deconvolve software. For spheres diffusing in a continuum medium at infinite dilution, in the approximation of spherical objects, the diffusion coefficient is related to the hydrodynamic radius, R_h, through the Stokes–Einstein equation:

$$R_h = \frac{kT}{6\pi\eta_0 D} \quad (2)$$

where k is the Boltzmann constant, T is the absolute temperature and $\eta_0 = 0.89 cP$ is the solvent viscosity. For not spherical particles, R_h represents the radius of a spherical aggregate with the same diffusion coefficient measured. In the present system, due to the high dilution, it is possible to consider the approximation that $\eta \cong \eta_0$, where η represents the solution viscosity. In this hypothesis, Equation (2) can be reasonably used to estimate the averaged hydrodynamic radius of the particles.

3.2. Synthetic Procedures and Characterization of Intermediates 4–7, (S)-1,2-O-Distearoyl Glycerol and Pure Sulfavant S (3)

Compound 4: Sodium hydride (0.235 g, 0.01 mol) was portion-wise added to (S)-(+)-1,2-isopropylideneglycerol (0.6 g, 0.00457 mol) dissolved in THF (7.5 mL), and after 30 min of stirring benzyl bromide (0.85 g, 0.005 mol) was added; after 20 h at 60 °C the mixture was evaporated and purified by silica gel chromatography using a light petroleum ether/diethyl ether gradient to give 4 (1.0 g, 0.0045 mol, 94%); ^{1}H-NMR (400 MHz, CDCl$_3$): δ 7.19–7.08 (5H, overlapped), 4.38 (2H, bs), 4.12 (1H, m), 3.86 (1H, m), 3.58 (1H, m), 3.38 (1H, m), 3.30 (1H, m), 1.27 (3H, s), 1.20 (3H, s); HRESIMS m/z 245.1140 [M + Na]$^+$ (calcd for C$_{13}$H$_{18}$O$_3$Na$^+$, 245.1148).

Compound 5: Compound 4 (1.0 g, 0.0045 mol) was dissolved in methanol/water 95/5 (7 mL) and Dowex H$^+$ (7.3 g) was added; after stirring for 1.5 h the mixture was filtered and evaporated giving compound 5 (0.762 g, 0.0042 mol, 93%); ^{1}H-NMR (400 MHz, CDCl$_3$): δ 7.29–7.17 (5H, overlapped, Ph), 4.58 (2H, bs), 3.86 (1H, m), 3.60 (1H, m), 3.52 (1H, m), 3.44 (2H, m); HRESIMS m/z 205.0829 [M + Na]$^+$ (calcd for C$_{10}$H$_{14}$O$_3$Na$^+$, 205.0835).

Compound 6: Compound 5 (0.762 g, 0.0042 mol) was dissolved in anhydrous dichloromethane (7 mL) before addition of 1.1 equiv. of stearic acid, N,N'-dicyclohexylcarbodiimide (1.0 g, 0.008 mol) and 4-dimethylaminopyridine (0.51 g, 0.0042 mol) under argon. The reaction mixture was stirred for 16 h at 25 °C; after evaporation under reduced pressure, the mixture was purified by silica gel chromatography using a gradient of petroleum ether/diethyl ether to give compound 6 (2.76 g, 0.0039 mol, 92%) as pale-yellow oil. ^{1}H-NMR (400 MHz, CDCl$_3$): δ 7.29–7.17 (5H, overlapped, Ph), 5.28, (1H, m, H-2), 4.57 (2H, CH$_2$Bn), 4.39 (1H, dd, = 3.76 and 11.8 Hz, H-1a), 4.23 (1H, dd, J = 6.4 and 11.8 Hz, H-1b), 3.63 (2H, bd, J = 5.2 Hz, H-3), 2.33 (4H, m, α-methylene), 1.63 (4H, m, β-methylene), 1.28–1,32 (56H, m, acyl chains CH$_2$), 0.83 (6H, overlapped, acyl chains CH$_3$); HRESIMS m/z 737.6062 [M + Na]$^+$ (calcd for C$_{46}$H$_{82}$O$_5$Na$^+$, 737.6054).

(S)-1,2-O-distearoyl glycerol: Compound 6 (2.76 g, 0.0039 mol) was dissolved in THF/MeOH 1/1 (25 mL) and Pd-C (10%) (0.350 g) was added; after stirring for 16 h at 25 °C the mixture was filtered, evaporated and purified by silica gel chromatography using a light petroleum ether/ethyl acetate gradient to give (S)-1,2-O-distearoyl glycerol (0.875 g, 0.0014 mol, 35%); ^{1}H-NMR (400 MHz, CDCl$_3$): δ 5.1 (1H, m, H-2), 4.32 (1H, dd, J = 4.4 and 11.9 Hz, H-1a), 4.23 (1H, dd, J = 5.8 and 11.9 Hz, H-1b), 3.72 (2H, bd, J = 4.8 Hz, H-3), 2.33 (4H, m, α-methylene), 1.63 (4H, m, β-methylene), 1.21–1.35 (56H, m, acyl chains CH$_2$), 0.85 (6H, overlapped, acyl chains CH$_3$); HRESIMS m/z 647.5591 [M + Na]$^+$ (calcd for C$_{39}$H$_{76}$O$_5$Na$^+$, 647.5585).

Compound 7: Peracetylated glucosyl-trichloroacetimidate (0.491 g, 0.001 mol) and (S)-1,2-O- distearoyl glycerol (0.625 g, 0.001 mol) were dissolved in anhydrous dichloromethane (15 mL), and the solution was kept at 0 °C; then, trimethylsilyl trifluoromethanesulfonate (TMSOTf) (35 μL in 1.5 mL of CH$_2$Cl$_2$) was added dropwise. The reaction mixture was stirred on activated 3 Å molecular sieves under argon for 5 h at 0 °C and quenched adding triethylamine (150 μL); after evaporation under reduced pressure the crude product was purified by silica gel chromatography using a gradient of petroleum ether/diethyl ether to give compound 7 (0.430 g, 0.00045 mol, 45%). ^{1}H-NMR (300 MHz, CDCl$_3$): δ 5.19 (1H, m), 5.06 (1H, overlapped), 4.99 (1H, t, J = 9.5 Hz), 4.88 (1H, dd, J = 9.5 and 7.9 Hz), 4.52 (1H, d), 4.02–4.32 (4H, overlapped), 3.93 (1H, dd, J = 11.0 and 4.9 Hz), 3.68 (2H, m), 2.3 (4H, m, α-methylenes) 1.98–2.02 (12H, bt), 1.60 (4H, m, β-methylenes), 1.32–1.22 (56H, acyl chains CH$_2$), 0.89 (6H, overlapped, acyl chains CH$_3$); HRESIMS m/z 977.6545 [M + Na]$^+$ (calcd for C$_{53}$H$_{94}$O$_{14}$Na, 977.6541).

Sulfavant S (3): white solid; ^{1}H-NMR (400 MHz, CD$_3$OD/CDCl$_3$ 1/1): δ values are referred to CHD$_2$OD (3.34 ppm and 49.0 ppm): δ 5.28 (1H, m, H-2), 4.40 (1H, dd, J = 2.7, 12.0 Hz, H-1a), 4.31 (1H, d, J = 7.6 H-1'), 4.24 (1H, dd, J = 6.9, 12.0 Hz, H-1b), 4.05 (1H, dd, J = 5.4, 11.0 Hz, H-3a), 3.79–3.71 (3H, H-3b, H-3', H-4'), 3.41 (1H, bt, J = 8.9 Hz, H-2'), 3.26 (1H, overlapped, H-6'a), 3.25 (1H, overlapped, H-5'), 3.09 (1H, dd, J = 7.2, 15.7 Hz, H-6'b), 2.36–2.27 (4H, α-methylenes of stearoyl portions), 1.65–1.56 (4H, β-methylenes of stearoyl portions), 1.36–1.20 (60H, aliphatic methylenes), 0.89 (6H, bt, J = 6.0 Hz, 2CH$_3$); ^{13}C-NMR (100MHz, CD$_3$OD:CDCl$_3$ 1:1): δ 174.1, 173.7 (C, acyl esters of stearoyl part), 103.2 (CH, C1'), 76.1 (CH, C2'), 73.8 (CH, C5'), 72.4 (CH, C3'), 72.3 (CH, C4'), 70.2 (CH, C2), 68.2 (CH$_2$, C3), 63.2 (CH$_2$, C1), 53.6 (CH$_2$, C6'), 34.2 (CH$_2$, α-methylene of stearoyl portion), 32.2–29.0 (CH$_2$, methylenes of stearoyl portion), 24.9 (CH$_2$, β-methylene of stearoyl portion), 13.8 (CH$_3$, methyls of stearoyl portion); HRESIMS m/z 849.5772 [M-K]$^-$ (calcd for C$_{45}$H$_{85}$O$_{12}$S$^-$, 849.5767).

3.3. Human Monocyte-Dendritic Cell Differentation

For each assay, human peripheral blood mononuclear cells were isolated from two healthy donors by standard Ficoll density gradient centrifugation. Monocytes were purified from human peripheral blood mononuclear cells using MACS CD14 microbeads (Miltenyi Biotech, Auburn, AL, USA) according to the manufacturer's recommendation. Purity was checked by staining with a FITC-conjugated anti-CD14 antibody (Milteny Biotech) and FACS analysis and was routinely found to be greater than 98%. Immature DCs were obtained by incubating monocytes at 1×10^6 cells mL^{-1} in an RPMI 1640 medium supplemented with 10% fetal calf serum, 1% L-glutamine 2mM, 1% penicillin and streptomycin, human IL-4 (5 ng/mL), and human GM-CSF (100 ng/mL) for five days.

3.4. Cells Staining and Stimulation

After five days in culture, surface staining was performed on monocyte-derived dendritic cells (moDCs) for flow cytometry analysis. moDCs (0.8×10^6 cell/well) were then incubated with synthetic compounds in 12 wells at the reported concentrations. Stimulation with PAM2CSK4 1 µg mL^{-1} (Invivogen) was used as positive control. After 24 h, expression of all surface markers was estimated by using the following conjugated mAbs from Miltenyi Biotec: HLA-DR FITC, CD83 PE and CD86 APC, and analyzed by a flow cytometer (BD ACCURI, BD Bioscience, Milano, Italy) according to standard protocol.

3.5. Statistical Analysis

All data were analyzed by one-way ANOVA, followed by the Tukey test for multiple comparisons. A *p*-value less than 0.05 was considered statistically significant. All analyses were performed using the GraphPad Prism 8.00 for Windows software (GraphPad Software, San Diego, CA, USA).

3.6. Characterization of Colloid Nanoparticles

After purification by HPLC, samples were prepared in 1 mL of Millipore water at 0.1 mM of each compound **1–3** and mixtures **2** and **3**. After sonication for 30 min at 35 °C, the solutions were maintained at room temperature (20 °C) for 24 h. The mean diffusion coefficients were obtained as an average of at least three measurements at 25 °C.

4. Conclusions

Sulfavants are bioactive molecules able to induce DC maturation and trigger an adaptive immune response in vivo [13–15]. The activity of these products is largely dependent on the formation of colloidal particles under aqueous conditions [12]. Mixing diastereoisomers **2** and **3**, both active at nanomolar concentrations in pure form, determined a consistent decrease of the biological response in agreement with formation of supramolecular aggregates of different size and stability. Multiple equilibria between free active monomers and different aggregates control the concentration of the products able to bind the cellular targets, thus affecting the results of biological tests and accuracy of the evaluation of the therapeutic potential. In our opinion, this behavior is common to many other lipophilic or amphiphilic compounds, such as natural products, lipopeptides and glycolipids, whose activity can be significantly altered by supramolecular self-assembly in aqueous media. This effect could be more relevant in in vitro assays than in vivo trials since the presence of proteins and other molecules in the body fluids can reduce the tendency of these compounds to aggregate. Sulfavant S (**3**) was synthesized by a modified protocol involving the preparation of (*S*)-1,2-*O*-distearoylglycerol as an alternative acceptor of the glucosyl-trichloroacetimidate donor. This approach allows to overcome the technical issues arising by the low stereocontrol of the coupling reaction and represents a starting point for the preparation of other members of this new family of immunomodulatory agents.

Author Contributions: E.M. and A.F. conceived and coordinated the study. L.F., M.Z., G.N. and G.D. carried out the experimental works and data analysis. L.F., A.B. and A.F. (Antonio Fabozzi) DLS analysis. R.D.P. and

C.G. performed biological tests. E.M. and A.F. (Angelo Fontana) wrote the manuscript with contributions of all coauthors. All authors have read and agreed to the published version of the manuscript.

Funding: This research was funded in the frame of the project ADViSE Antitumor Drugs and Vaccines from the SEa approved by Campania with D.D 403 of 12/11/2018 and integration D.D: n.422 of 16/11/2018.

Acknowledgments: E.M. and A.F. thank BioSEArch SRL for the generous support; moreover, the authors wish to thank European Union (FSE, PON Ricerca e Innovazione 2014–2020, Azione I.1 "Dottorati Innovativi con caratterizzazione Industriale") for funding a Ph.D. grant to one of the authors (Laura Fioretto).

Conflicts of Interest: The authors declare no conflict of interest.

References

1. Lehn, J.M. Toward self-organization and complex matter. *Science* **2002**, *295*, 2400–2403. [CrossRef] [PubMed]
2. Waring, M.J. Lipophilicity in drug discovery. *Expert Opin. Drug Discov.* **2010**, *5*, 235–248. [CrossRef] [PubMed]
3. Aguilar, J.C.; Rodríguez, E.G. Vaccine adjuvants revisited. *Vaccine* **2007**, *25*, 3752–3762. [CrossRef]
4. Xu, F.; Valiante, N.M.; Ulmer, J.B. Small molecule immunopotentiators as vaccine adjuvants. In *Vaccine Adjuvants and Delivery Systems*; Singh, M., Ed.; John Wiley & Sons, Inc.: Hoboken, NJ, USA, 2007; pp. 175–189.
5. Egli, A.; Santer, D.M.; Barakat, K.; Zand, M.; Levin, A.; Vollmer, M.; Weisser, M.; Khanna, N.; Kumar, D.; Tyrrell, D.L.; et al. Vaccine adjuvants—Understanding molecular mechanisms to improve vaccines. *Swiss Med. Wkly.* **2014**, *144*, w13940. [CrossRef] [PubMed]
6. De Gregorio, E.; D'Oro, U.; Wack, A. Immunology of TLR-independent vaccine adjuvants. *Curr. Opin. Immunol.* **2009**, *21*, 339–345. [CrossRef]
7. Wu, T.Y.-H.; Singh, M.; Miller, A.T.; De Gregorio, E.; Doro, F.; D'Oro, U.; Skibinski, D.A.G.; Mbow, M.L.; Bufali, S.; Herman, A.E.; et al. Rational design of small molecules as vaccine adjuvants. *Sci. Transl. Med.* **2014**, *6*, 263ra160. [CrossRef]
8. De Gregorio, E.; Rappuoli, R. From empiricism to rational design: A personal perspective of the evolution of vaccine development. *Nat. Rev. Immunol.* **2014**, *14*, 505–514. [CrossRef]
9. Johnson, D.A.; Baldridge, J.R. TLR4 Agonists as vaccine adjuvants. In *Vaccine Adjuvants and Delivery Systems*; Singh, M., Ed.; John Wiley & Sons, Inc.: Hoboken, NJ, USA, 2007; pp. 131–156.
10. Reed, S.G.; Orr, M.T.; Fox, C.B. Key roles of adjuvants in modern vaccine. *Nat. Med.* **2013**, *19*, 1597–1608. [CrossRef]
11. Garcon, N.; Di Pasquale, A. From discovery to licensure, the Adjuvant System story. *Human Vaccines Immunother.* **2017**, *13*, 19–33. [CrossRef]
12. Manzo, E.; Gallo, C.; Fioretto, L.; Nuzzo, G.; Barra, G.; Pagano, D.; Russo Krauss, I.; Paduano, L.; Ziaco, M.; DellaGreca, M.; et al. Diasteroselective colloidal self-assembly affects the immunological response of the molecular adjuvant Sulfavant. *ACS Omega* **2019**, *4*, 7807–7814. [CrossRef]
13. Manzo, E.; Cutignano, A.; Pagano, D.; Gallo, C.; Barra, G.; Nuzzo, G.; Sansone, C.; Ianora, A.; Urbanek, K.; Fenoglio, D.; et al. A new marine-derived sulfoglycolipid triggers dendritic cell activation and immune adjuvant response. *Sci. Rep.* **2017**, *7*, 6286. [CrossRef] [PubMed]
14. Manzo, E.; Fioretto, L.; Pagano, D.; Nuzzo, G.; Gallo, C.; De Palma, R.; Fontana, A. Chemical synthesis of marine-derived sulfoglycolipids, a new class of molecular adjuvants. *Mar. Drugs* **2017**, *15*, 288. [CrossRef] [PubMed]
15. Manzo, E.; Ciavatta, M.L.; Pagano, D.; Fontana, A. An efficient and versatile chemical synthesis of bioactive glycoglycerolipids. *Tetrahedron Lett.* **2012**, *53*, 879–881. [CrossRef]
16. Mellman, I. Dendritic cells: Master regulators of the immune response. *Cancer Immunol. Res.* **2013**, *1*, 145–149. [CrossRef] [PubMed]
17. Pearce, E.J.; Everts, B. Dendritic cell metabolism. *Nat. Rev. Immunol.* **2015**, *15*, 18–29. [CrossRef]
18. Sallusto, F.; Lanzavecchia, A. Efficient Presentation of Soluble Antigen by Cultured Human Dendritic Cells Is Maintained by Granulocyte/Macrophage Colony-stimulating Factor Plus Iuterleukin 4 and Downregulated by Tumor Necrosis Factor α. *J. Exp. Med.* **1994**, *179*, 1109–1118. [CrossRef] [PubMed]
19. Rossi, M.; Young, J.W. Human Dendritic Cells: Potent Antigen-Presenting Cells at the Crossroads of Innate and Adaptive Immunity. *J. Immunol.* **2005**, *175*, 1373–1381. [CrossRef]

20. Hart, D.N.J. Dendritic Cells: Unique Leukocyte Populations Which Control the Primary Immune Response. *J. Am. Soc. Hematol* **1997**, *90*, 3245–3287. [CrossRef]
21. Guermonprez, P.; Valladeau, J.; Zitvogel, L.; Théry, C.; Amigorena, S. Antigen presentation and T Cell stimulation by Dendritic Cells. *Annu. Rev. Immunol.* **2002**, *20*, 621–677. [CrossRef]
22. Lanzavecchia, A.; Sallusto, F. Regulation of T cell immunity by Dendritic cells. *Cell* **2001**, *106*, 263–266. [CrossRef]
23. Steinman, R.M.; Hemmi, H. Dendritic cells: Translating innate to adaptive immunity. *Curr. Top. Microbiol. Immunol.* **2006**, *311*, 17–58. [PubMed]
24. Steinman, R.M.; Pope, M. Exploiting dendritic cells to improve vaccine efficacy. *J. Clin. Invest.* **2002**, *109*, 1519–1526. [CrossRef] [PubMed]
25. Kastenmüller, W.; Kastenmüller, K.; Kurts, C.; Seder, R.A. Dendritic cell-targeted vaccines—Hope or hype? *Nat. Rev. Immunol.* **2014**, *14*, 705–711. [CrossRef] [PubMed]
26. Palucka, K.; Banchereau, J. Cancer immunotherapy via dendritic cells. *Nat. Rev. Cancer* **2012**, *12*, 265–277. [CrossRef]
27. Zhou, L.J.; Tedder, T.F. Human blood dendritic cells selectively express CD83, a member of the immunoglobulin superfamily. *J. Immunol.* **1995**, *154*, 3821–3835.
28. Owen, S.C.; Doak, A.K.; Ganesh, A.N.; Nedyalkova, L.; McLaughlin, C.K.; Shoichet, B.K.; Shoichet, M.S. Colloidal drug formulations can explain "bell-shaped" concentration-response curves. *ACS Chem. Biol.* **2014**, *9*, 777–784. [CrossRef]
29. Matsumoto, K.; Sakai, H.; Takeuchi, R.; Tsuchiya, K.; Ohta, K.; Sugawara, F.; Abe, M.; Sakaguchi, K. Effective form of sulfoquinovosyldiacyglycerol (SQDG) vesicles for DNA polymerase inhibition. *Colloids Surfaces B Biointerfaces* **2005**, *46*, 175–181. [CrossRef]
30. Yamamoto, Y.; Sahara, H.; Takenouchi, M.; Matsumoto, Y.; Imai, A.; Fujita, T.; Tamura, Y.; Takahashi, N.; Gasa, S.; Matsumoto, K.; et al. Inhibition of CD62L+T-cell response in vitro via a novel sulfo-glycolipid, β-SQAG9 liposome that binds to CD62L molecule on the cell surface. *Cell. Immunol.* **2004**, *232*, 105–115. [CrossRef]
31. Aoki, S.; Ohta, K.; Matsumoto, K.; Sakai, H.; Abe, M.; Miura, M.; Sugawara, F.; Sakaguchi, K. An emulsion of sulfoquinovosylacylglycerol with long-chain alkanes increases its permeability to tumor cells. *J. Membr. Biol.* **2006**, *213*, 11–18. [CrossRef]
32. Matsumoto, K.; Takenouchi, M.; Ohta, K.; Ohta, Y.; Imura, T.; Oshige, M.; Yamamoto, Y.; Sahara, H.; Sakai, H.; Abe, M.; et al. Design of vesicles of 1,2-di-O-acyl-3-O-(β-D-sulfoquinovosyl)-glyceride bearing two stearic acids (β-SQDG-C18), a novel immunosuppressive drug. *Biochem. Pharmacol.* **2004**, *68*, 2379–2386. [CrossRef]

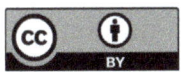

© 2020 by the authors. Licensee MDPI, Basel, Switzerland. This article is an open access article distributed under the terms and conditions of the Creative Commons Attribution (CC BY) license (http://creativecommons.org/licenses/by/4.0/).

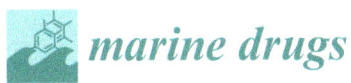

Article

Expression of Genes Related to Carrageenan Synthesis during Carposporogenesis of the Red Seaweed *Grateloupia imbricata*

Pilar Garcia-Jimenez *, Sara R. Mantesa and Rafael R. Robaina

Departamento de Biología, Facultad de Ciencias del Mar, Instituto de Estudios Ambientales y Recursos Naturales, Universidad de Las Palmas de Gran Canaria, E-35017 Las Palmas de Gran Canaria, Spain; saramantesa@gmail.com (S.R.M.); rafael.robaina@ulpgc.es (R.R.R.)
* Correspondence: pilar.garcia@ulpgc.es

Received: 22 July 2020; Accepted: 18 August 2020; Published: 19 August 2020

Abstract: Carrageenan, the foremost constituent of extracellular matrix of some rhodophyta, is a galactan backbone with a different number of sulphate groups attached. Variations of degree of sulphation are associated with different types of carrageenans, which vary according to seaweed life cycles, and have consequences for the exploitation of this raw material. In this work, we used three well-recognised stages of development thalli and two stages of cystocarp maturation to analyse genes that encode addition and elimination of sulphate groups to cell-wall galactan of the red seaweed *Grateloupia imbricata*. Expressions of *carbohydrate sulfotransferase* and *galactose-6 sulfurylase* and genes encoding stress proteins such as cytochrome P450 and WD40, were examined. Results showed that transcript expression of *carbohydrate sulfotransferase* occurs at all stage of thalli development. Meanwhile *galactose-6 sulfurylase* expressions displayed different roles, which could be related to a temporal regulation of cystocarp maturation. *Cytochrome P450* and *WD40* are related to the disclosure and maturation of cystocarps of *G. imbricata*. Our conclusion is that differential expression of genes encoding proteins involved in the sulphation and desulphation of galactan backbone is associated with alterations in thalli development and cystocarp maturation in the red seaweed *Grateloupia imbricata*. Exploitation of industry-valued carrageenan will depend on insight into gene mechanisms of red seaweeds.

Keywords: carbohydrate sulfotransferase; carrageenan; cytochrome P450; galactose-6 sulfurylase; red alga; reproduction stages; WD 40

1. Introduction

Red seaweed cell-walls are mainly made of complex sulphated galactans primarily agar and carrageenans, which comprise a large family of hydrocolloids, depending on the varying degree of sulphation [1–3]. Specifically, carrageenans can be classified according to their gel-forming ability [4]. The differences among the various forms of carrageenan (κ-, ι- and λ-carrageenans) are related to the amount of sulphate groups, affecting solubility in water and the strength of carrageenans [5]. Moreover, cell walls have to change their carrageenan composition to adapt to the different development stages of the seaweed [6]. Thus, carragenophytic-alga gametophytes are known to be composed of κ- and ι carrageenan, whereas tetrasporophytes have λ-carrageenan [4].

Seaweed responses to the presence of reproductive structures is to push thallus cells to the sides, generate anatomical changes to locate reproductive structures and trigger fluctuations in the composition of the cell wall [4,7]. As the integrity of the cell wall is essential for maintaining growth and development of alga thalli and for the survival of reproductive structures, alterations in carrageenan composition can be assumed, as galactose units work together to build, incorporate and remove sulphated groups to and from the growing strands of galactans. Furthermore, these changes in the amount of sulphate groups influence the ability of seaweed to model responses, such as the softening and flexibility of thalli and facilitating the growth in size of reproductive structures. Seaweed can also display responses for recovering of thallus status after sporogenesis.

Additionally, sporogenesis is inherently linked to stressors such as volatile growth regulators, tide periods, hours of irradiation and temperature [8–10]. These environmental stressors also have an impact on generating reactive oxygen species (ROS in the form of O_2, H_2O_2 or OH^-) [9,10]. Moreover, ROSs also play an important role in softening thalli and therefore also facilitate the development of cystocarps in red seaweed [8]. Reactive oxygen species act as signalling molecules under stress and induce cell responses [11,12]. Moreover proteins, such as WD40 and cytochrome P450, can be synthesised to reduce such oxidative damage [9,10,13]. Carrageenans, as components of the cell wall in seaweeds, have been reported to also show antioxidant activity by scavenging hydrogen peroxide [14,15].

Consistent with the chemical complexity of the cell wall and multiple environment stressors, the transcriptional machinery underlying synthesis and modification of cell-wall polysaccharides is intricate. Particularly in the case of carrageenans, the biosynthesis pathway has not been fully described, although three main classes of enzymes have been proposed namely galactosyltransferases, sulfotransferases and galactose 6 sulfurylases [16]. Significantly, carbohydrate sulfotransferase, which add a sulphate group from a donor molecule (often 3′phosphoadenosine-5′phosphosulfate, PAPS), have been described in carrageenophytes. Galactose-6 sulfurylase, which catalyses the formation of the 3,6-anhydrogalactose residues by removing C6 sulphate group in sulphated galactans [17], has also been reported specifically in red macroalgae (Figure 1).

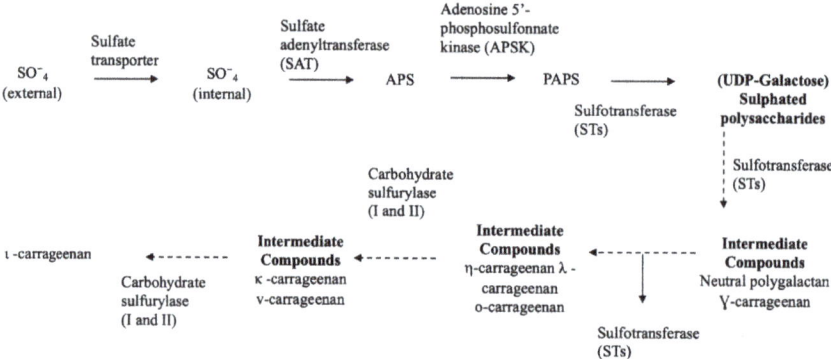

Figure 1. Schematic biosynthetic pathway for sulphate assimilation and synthesis of carrageenan. PAPS, 3′phosphoadenosine-5′phosphosulfate.

Grateloupia imbricata is a carragenophytic red seaweed, with triphasic life cycle (Figure 2). This macroalga represents a candidate model organism for basic studies of physiology, owing to its ability to produce raw material such as carrageenan.

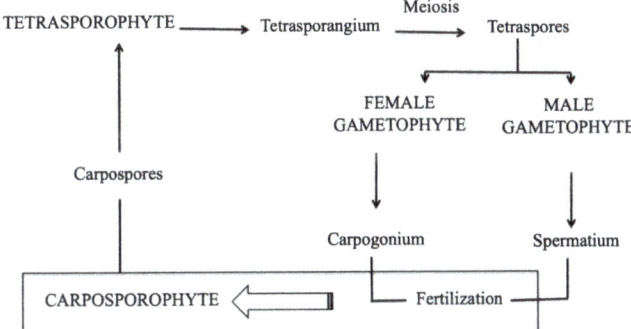

Figure 2. Diagram of a tri-genetic life cycle in the red alga *Grateloupia imbricata* comprising gametophytes (haploids), the carposporophyte, that develops on the female gametophyte after fertilisation, and the sporophyte (diploid). Taken from Garcia-Jimenez and Robaina (2019) DOI: http://dx.doi.org/10.5772/intechopen.83353.

Transcriptome information of *G. imbricata* revealed the presence of transcripts required for biosynthesis of sulphated polysaccharides, so the study of these transcripts can contribute to the understanding of carrageenan synthesis [18]. This paper focuses on the characterisation of expression of genes such as *carbohydrate sulfotransferase* and *galactose 6 sulfurylase* that are specifically related to addition and removal of sulphate groups to galactan. We hypothesised that the expression of genes encoding enzymes of carrageenan synthesis in *G. imbricata* can be a starting point for further studies on sulphation of carrageenan. Moreover, these genes can be correlated to reproductive stage (carposporogenesis) of *G. imbricata*. Our aim is to show that the expression of two genes involved in the sulphation (*carbohydrate sulfotransferase*) and desulphation (*galactose-6 sulfurylase*) of the galactan backbone is related to the stage of development of thalli and to reproductive structures (cystocarps) through flexibility and softening of thalli. Likewise, we determine to what extent genes encoding stress proteins (*Cytochrome P450* and *WD 40*) can also be involved during cystocarp maturation, as the presence of cystocarps would also comprise the cell wall softening.

2. Results

To determine the sulphation and desulphation of galactan, transcript expressions of *carbohydrate sulfotransferase* in charge of addition sulphate groups and *galactose-6 sulfurylase* for removing sulphate groups were determined according to development stage of thalli and to the presence of reproductive structures (cystocarps; Figure 3).

2.1. Gene Expression for Stages of Thalli Development

Expression levels of each of two gene sequences encoding *sulfotransferase* and *sulfurylase* for infertile, fertilised and fertile thalli are shown (Figure 4). Expressions for *sulfotransferase*, *ST1* and *ST2*, exhibit similar behaviour (Figure 4A). In addition, no significative differences in levels of expression are reported between different stages of development of the thalli (Figure 4A).

Different transcript expressions are shown for *sulfurylase* depending on the development stage of the thalli. Thus, when transcript expression for *sulfurylase 1* (*SY1*) was compared to that of infertile thalli, *SY1* was overexpressed for fertilised thalli and down expressed for fertile thalli (Figure 4B). Meanwhile the transcript expression for *SY2* was significantly down-expressed for fertilised and fertile thalli, compared to infertile thalli (Figure 4B). Significant differential expression is also reported when *sulfurylase SY1* and *SY2* from fertilised thalli are compared.

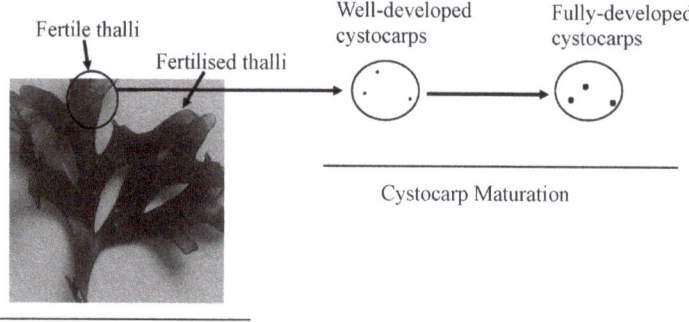

Figure 3. Schematic showing different development stages of thalli (fertilised and fertile thalli) and cystocarps maturation (well-developed and fully-developed cystocarps) of *Grateloupia imbricata*. Infertile thalli are thalli without cystocarps in all axes of the same individual.

2.2. Gene Expression for the Maturation of Reproductive Structures (Cystocarps)

Expression levels of *sulfotransferase* (*ST1* and *ST2*) in the presence of fully-developed cystocarps show significant over-expression compared to the absence of cystocarps and well-developed cystocarps (Figure 5A,B).

Regarding *sulfurylase*, expression levels of *SY1* and *SY2* show different behaviours. On the one hand, *sulfurylase SY1* is over-expressed in well-developed cystocarps in comparison with fully-developed cystocarps (Figure 6A).

On the other hand, *sulfurylase SY2* is expressed significantly in the presence of fully-developed cystocarps. Thus, this expression was related to the maturity of the cystocarps (Figure 6B).

2.3. Gene Expression Encoding Stress Proteins during Cystocarp Maturation

Levels of the expression of *Cytochrome P450* and *WD 40* follow a similar pattern (Figure 7). No significant differences were found in the *Cytochrome P450* and *WD 40* expression levels in thalli with well-developed cystocarps when compared to those without cystocarps (dotted line, Figure 7). The gene transcript expression is only significant for *WD40* in fully-developed cystocarps in comparison with well-developed cystocarps (Figure 7).

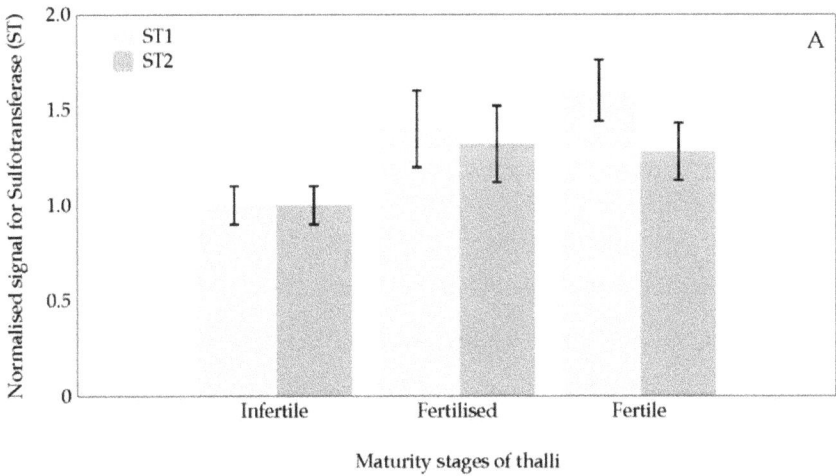

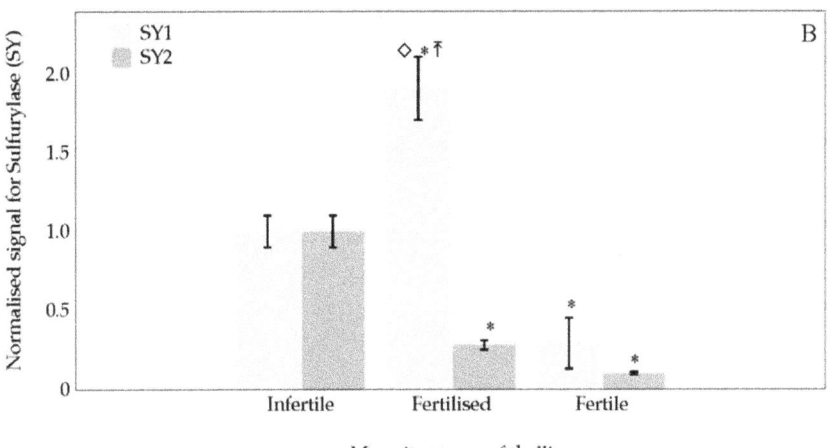

Figure 4. Normalised expression signal during three thalli development stages (infertile, fertilised and fertile thalli) of *Grateloupia imbricata* for (**A**) two *carbohydrate sulfotransferase* (*Sulfotransferase*, *ST1* and *ST2*); (**B**) two *galactose-6 sulfurylase* (*Sulfurylase SY1* and *SY2*). Data in bars are the mean ± SD, $n = 4$. Different symbols mean significant differences ($p < 0.01$) between infertile thalli and fertilised and fertile thalli (*), between two gene sequences 1 and 2 (↤), and between different stages of development (◇).

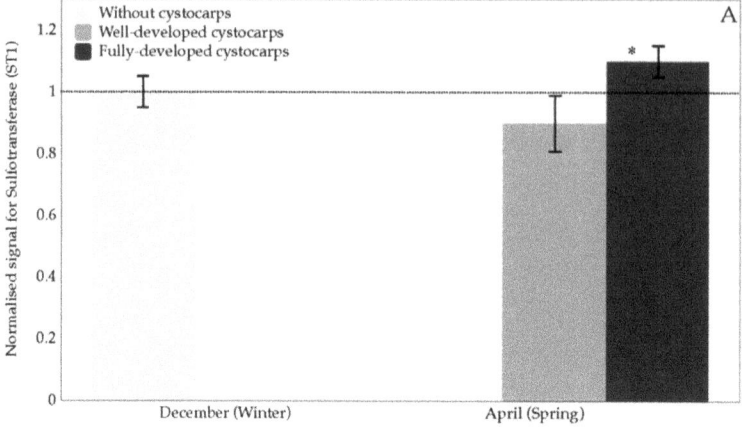

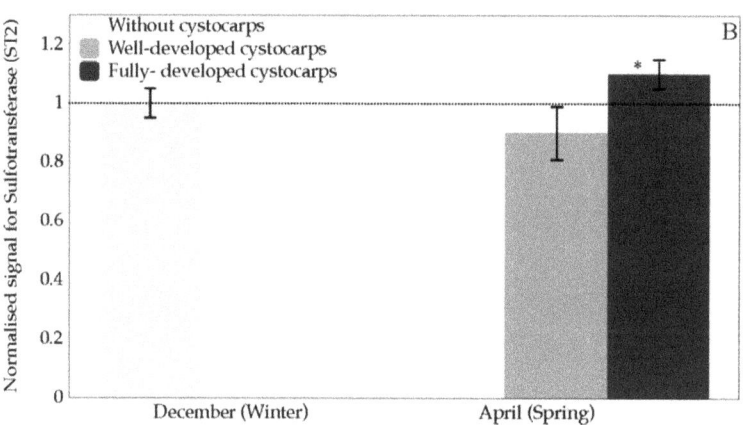

Figure 5. Normalised expression for *carbohydrate sulfotransferase* during two stages of cystocarps maturation (well-developed and fully-developed cystocarps) of *Grateloupia imbricata* for (**A**) *Sulfotransferase, ST1*; (**B**) *Sulfotransferase, ST2*. Data in bars are the mean ± SD, $n = 4$. * significant differences ($p < 0.01$) between samples without cystocarps and at different maturation stages. Dotted line corresponds to transcript expression from pooled thalli containing cystocarps at different stages of development and thalli without cystocarps ($n = 8$).

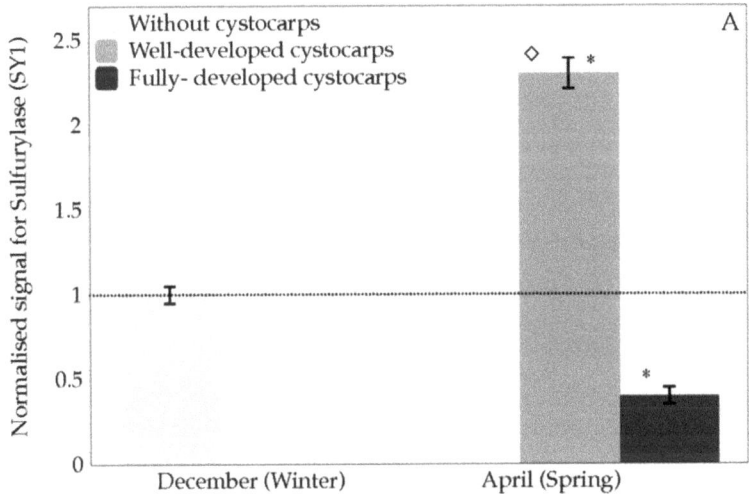

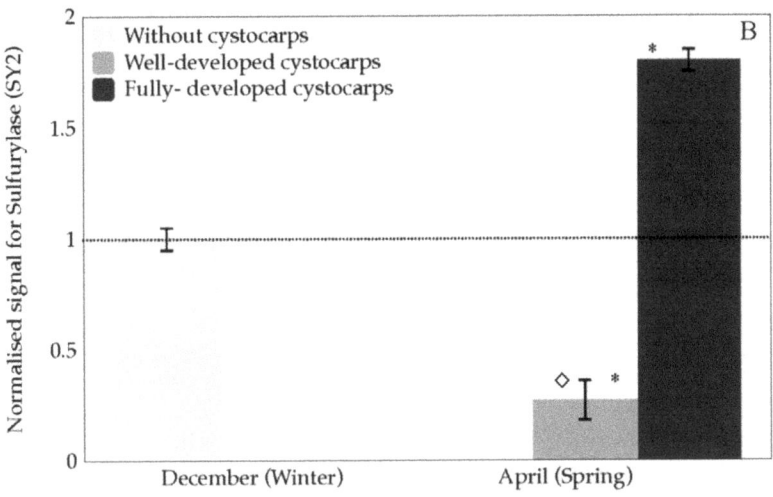

Figure 6. Normalised expression for *galactose-6 sulfurylase* during two stages of cystocarps maturation (well-developed and fully-developed cystocarps) of *Grateloupia imbricata* for (**A**) *Sulfurylase SY1*; (**B**) *Sulfurylase SY2*. Data in bars are the mean ± SD, $n = 4$. Different symbols mean significant differences ($p < 0.01$) between samples without cystocarps and at different maturation stages (*), and between different stages of cystocarps maturation for the same gene (◊). Dotted line corresponds to transcript expression from pooled thalli containing cystocarps at different stages of development and thalli without cystocarps ($n = 8$).

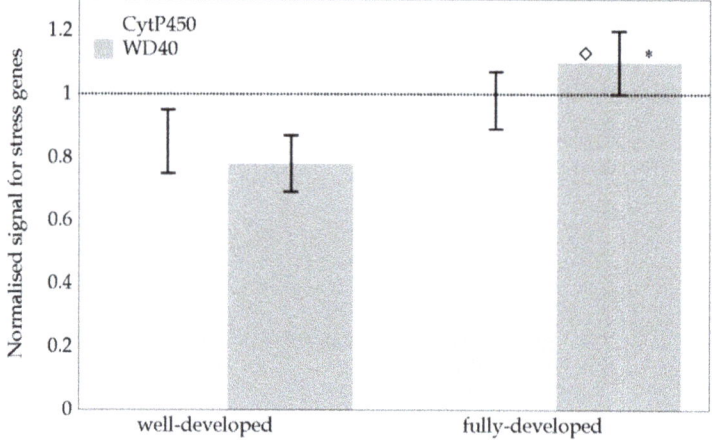

Figure 7. Normalised expression for *Cytochrome P450* and *WD40* during two stages of cystocarps maturation (well-developed and fully-developed cystocarps) of *Grateloupia imbricata* Data in bars are the mean ± SD, $n = 4$. Different symbols mean significant differences ($p < 0.01$) between thalli with cystocarps and those without them (*), and between different stages of cystocarps maturation for the same gene (◊). Dotted line corresponds to gene transcript expression of thalli without cystocarps ($n = 8$).

3. Discussion

Seaweed cell-wall is made of different components namely cellulose, xylan, mannan, among others [19], although important constituents are alginates and fucans for brown algae, ulvans and other sulphated glycans for green algae, and agar and carrageenan for red algae [20]. The latter complex group of components are also sulphated polysaccharides which are recognised by their pharmacological and industrial uses [21]. In Rhodophyta, agar and carrageenan account for 40–50% of the dry weight, but can be as much as 70–80% [20]. Focusing on carrageenans, the backbone structure comprises linear chains of repeating D-galactose sugars and 3,6-anhydro-galactose units, with a different number and location of the sulphate groups attached. Sulphation degree and molecular conformation allow classifying carrageenans in three main types with commercial importance, namely κ-, ι- and λ-carrageenan, all containing 15–40% ester sulphate; although seaweeds can also contain hybrids carrageenans [22]. Sulphation takes place in the cell wall by the action of carbohydrate sulfotransferase whilst desulphation by galactose-6 sulfurylase also occurs in the cell wall, although its role is not fully clarified. Galactose-6 sulfurylase catalyses the conversion of μ-carrageenan into κ-carrageenan, but λ-carrageenan seems to not be susceptible to its action [16,23,24]. The number of sulphate groups is, in turn, one of the features that affects the properties of carrageenan types as carrageenans are gel-forming and viscosifying polysaccharides [25]. In addition, variations in carrageenan composition, i.e., sulphation degree, have been associated to life cycles stages of algae, alga species and environment conditions.

With the goal of revealing changes in sulphation degree of galactan of carrageenan during carposporogenesis in *G. imbricata*, expression levels of two genes involved in the biosynthesis of carrageenan has been reported. One of main achievements of this work lies on the fact that changes in transcript levels of these genes, i.e., *carbohydrate sulfotransferase* and *galactose-6-sulfurylase*, are associated at different stages of thalli development and the well-recognised stages of cystocarp maturation. Thus, expressions of *sulfotransferase* were reported in all stages of thalli development (Figure 4A). Results indicated that (1) the *ST1* and *ST2* could encode proteins responsible for similar mechanisms and metabolic pathways during thalli development, and (2) *sulfotransferase* could be involved in housekeeping activity as sulphated galactan is component of cell wall of red seaweeds. Hence, transcript expression suggests that the addition of sulphate groups occurs during all stages of thalli development.

It is also worth drawing attention to the behaviour of both *sulfurylase* sequences (Figure 4B). The expression behaviour of *sulfurylase* (*SY1* and *SY2*) indicated that they may play several roles and that they are time-regulated. It was also evident that *SY1* was induced to a larger extent when the thalli were fertilised (Figure 4B). Noticeably, overexpression was higher in *sulfurylase SY1* than *sulfurylase SY2* for fertilised thalli, suggesting a concrete development-specific expression role for the *sulfurylase SY1* gene during thalli maturation. Apart from that, *sulfurylase SY2* expressions may also depend on the stage of the thalli, as differential transcript expression was also reported, albeit with different expression levels that were significantly lower than those for *sulfurylase SY1* (Figure 4B). The exhibition of these expression patterns for *SY1* and *SY2* in the red seaweed *G. imbricata* opens up an interesting pathway for determining whether the differential expressions of *SY1* and *SY2* could be a consequence of specific transcription factors of each gene copy. Interestingly, it could infer the presence of specific transcription factors, which would only function efficiently at specific stages of thalli maturation. Hence, the different stages of seaweed thalli development could contribute to the expression of different regulatory proteins. In higher plants, different proteins can participate as elements of regulatory mechanisms and co-ordinate cell activity [26]. Furthermore, if the transcription factors were activated and regulatory proteins were synthesised, this would reinforce the theory of a time-gene regulation of two sulfurylase as thalli development proceeds. All in all, genes that encode proteins responsible for the desulphation of the galactan skeleton of the cell wall will allow *G. imbricata* thalli to soften and enable the development of reproductive structures (cystocarps) in thalli.

Cystocarp disclosure is elicited by complex multiple factors, encompassing the period from when cystocarps first become visible (well-developed cystocarps), through to the adequate development of cystocarps (fully-developed cystocarps). Thus, cystocarps could achieve optimal maturity when elicitation factors and the mechanisms that weaken and soften the cell wall act in co-ordination [8]. In line with this, the behaviour of the genes that encode the adding and elimination of the sulphate group during maturation of reproductive structures must be appraised, along with the genes that encode oxidative-stress-related proteins, which also potentially contribute to softening the thallus.

Little has been reported to date about genes that control sulphate addition. This is one of the few studies aimed at characterising *sulfotransferase* expression levels at different stages of maturity in red seaweed cystocarps. Although monitoring the expressions of two types of *sulfotransferase* (*ST1* and *ST2*) showed similar behaviour and transcript expression levels, significant transcript expression was shown in fully-developed cystocarps of *G. imbricata* (Figure 5A,B). Our results seem to suggest that genes encoding proteins that add the sulphate group are working to reconstitute the cell wall after disclosure and maturity of cystocarps and even early release of spores, as this is an unsynchronised process. Thus, it would not be misconceived to think that once fertilisation has occurred in *G. imbricata*, the re-arrangement of carrageenan constituents proceeds to improve and recover the organisation of the cell wall.

Remarkably, what occurs with *sulfurylase* differs from the expected. Following the line of argument, the thalli would soften prior to the appearance of cystocarps. Hence, one would expect transcript overexpression of *sulfurylase* to be reported when cystocarps are first developing (well-developed cystocarps) and always prior to their complete maturity (fully-developed cystocarps). However, *SY2* showed transcript expression is significantly higher in the presence of fully-developed cystocarps than in thalli with well-developed cystocarps (Figure 6B). Thus, different functionality of *SY1* and *SY2* can be assumed. To gain greater insight into what could be occurring, it is worth considering that fertilisation in *G. imbricata* takes place when a spermatium fertilises a carpogonium on the female gametophyte. The fertilised carpogonium develops into a structure called a cystocarp that will contain spores [27]. This cystocarp develops in the auxiliary ampulla after the auxiliary cell receives the diploid nuclei from the fertilised carpogonial cell [28]. Thus, carrying the argument of *SY* different functionality a step further, *SY1* may be responsible for weakening the cell wall to embrace the development of auxiliary ampulla cells, and *SY2* allows the cystocarps to grow in size and develop their spores within. These differentiated functions should show a co-ordination of the different kinds of *sulfurylase* over time and cell type during the cystocarp maturation. In short, this time–transcript expression could orchestrate specific adaptation and protective responses during cystocarps development. This would mean that *sulfurylase* genes are closely related to reproductive development and that maturity stages of cystocarps require genes expressed in different ways from early stages.

Beyond the sulphation and de-sulphation of galactan backbone as a consequence of thalli development and cystocarp maturation, the gene encoding *WD40* has also been reported to potentially play a role in cystocarp maturing, as the gene transcripts were significantly overexpressed in fully-developed cystocarps, compared with expression in developing cystocarps (Figure 7). To some extent, these results are to be expected as earlier studies on gene expression during carposporogenesis of *G. imbricata* showed *WD40* and *cytochrome P450* transcript expressions are limited to different signals related to both cystocarp disclosure and development of the red seaweed *G. imbricata* [9,10]. Specifically, *WD40* plays an active role in the processes of regulation and response to damage [29], so *WD40* gene expression in *G. imbricata* could suggest cross talk between cystocarp maturation and a reduction of oxidative damage.

In summary, gene expressions involved in the sulphation and desulphation of galactan backbone are associated with alterations in thalli development and cystocarp maturation in the red seaweed *G. imbricata*. This opens an interesting framework to gain insight into gene mechanisms involved in carrageenan synthesis.

4. Materials and Methods

4.1. Alga Material

Thalli from *G. imbricata* were collected along the northeast coast of Gran Canaria in the Canary Islands. Within 2 h of collection, thalli were examined under a stereomicroscope to identify cystocarps. Axes with no visible cystocarps (henceforth, fertilised thalli) and axes with light-red dots that are indicative of cystocarps (henceforth, fertile thalli), both belonging to the same individual (i.e., anchored to the same basal structure), were identified and separated for further use.

Two categories of fertile thalli were also identified; thalli with well-developed cystocarps and those that have fully-developed cystocarps (intense red dot and referred to as mature; Figure 3). Infertile thalli without any cystocarps were used as controls.

4.2. RNA Extraction

Total RNA from *G. imbricata* samples was isolated, as previously described [30]. In short, total RNA was extracted separately from the apical regions (100 mg) of fertilised, fertile, and infertile *G. mbricate* thalli using 1 mL of Tri-Reagent (Sigma, St. Louis, MO, USA) pursuant to the manufacturer's instructions. The isolated RNA samples were suspended individually in 20 µL of 1 M Tris-HCl, pH 8, 0.5 M EDTA and treated with DNase (1 U mg^{-1}; Promega, Madison, WI, USA) to destroy contaminating DNA. Total RNA was quantified in a TrayCell cuvette using a Beckman Coulter DU 530 spectrophotometer.

RNA (~1 µg from each sample) was reverse transcribed to first strand cDNA using an iScript Select cDNA Synthesis Kit (Bio-Rad; Hercules, CA, USA). The reverse transcriptase reaction was performed at 25 °C for 5 min, 42 °C for 30 min, and 85 °C for 5 min. The integrity of the cDNA was validated using a Nanodrop spectrophotometer (ThermoFisher Scientific, Waltham, MA, USA). The products were kept at 4 °C until used.

4.3. Quantitative Gene Expression

Before assaying for gene expression, a temperature gradient protocol was implemented for each set of primers to establish the best experimental conditions. The efficiency of the amplification and primer–dimer formation was assessed using a melting curve.

Real-time PCR was performed using SYBR Green master mix (Bio-Rad) and a forward and reverse primer pair (Table 1). Primers were designed from cDNA sequences of the *G. imbricata* transcriptome (BioProject record PRJNA309128). cDNA (2.5 µL) from apical parts of thalli in different maturity stages were used as a template. Real time PCR reactions were carried out with four replicates of each sample in a real-time PCR MiniOpticon thermal cycler (Bio-Rad) using the following steps: initial denaturation at 98 °C for 1 min, amplification during 30 cycles at the pertinent temperature for 1 min (Table 1), 72 °C for 5 min, followed by a final extension at 72 °C for 10 min.

All gene expressions were normalised using methods to validate potential constitutive genes along with the GenNorm basic visual application following calculations described in [31]. Five housekeeping genes were selected and tested, as previously described [32]. Two of the five constituent genes were validated as housekeeping genes that encode a large subunit of ribosomal RNA and the elongation factor 1α. We used amplicons (~70 nt) selected from conserved regions of the large subunit of the ribosomal RNA of *Grateloupia turuturu* (DQ364073), *Halymenia schizymenioid* (DQ364067) and *Cryptonemia undulata* (AF419133) and from the elongation factor of *Chondrus crispus* (CO653259) and *Haematococcus pluvialis* (DV203478) to follow the expression of genes. Data were represented as relative to the expression in infertile thalli and were expressed as the mean ± SD from four separate experiments.

Table 1. Sequences of the forward (F) and reverse (R) primers, and temperature of annealing (Tm) for each gene: *Carbohydrate sulfotransferase* (*ST1* and *ST2*), *Galactose-6 sulfurylase* (*SY1* and *SY2*), *WD 40* and *Cytochrome P450*.

Contig from *Grateloupia imbricata* Transcriptome	Primer Name		Sequence (5'-3')	Tm (°C)
3064	Carbohydrate sulfotransferase (ST1)	F	GCACCAAACGGCCACTAAAG	51
		R	AGGCGTTTTGTGATCTCCGA	
3265	Carbohydrate sulfotransferase (ST2)	F	GGGGACAAGACTGCGTTACA	51
		R	GAGATTGCGCATTCCGAACC	
137	galactose-6 sulfurylase (SY1)	F	CCCCAGTAGAAACGCGTGAT	55
		R	GACACCAAGAGTCCACCTCG	
824	galactose-6 sulfurylase (SY2)	F	GACAGCTTCGGTCTAGGAGC	55
		R	GGTGCAGGTCTTGCGTATCT	
10,134	WD40	F	GGCGCACATCCCAATACTT	52
		R	CTATCAACGCTCTCGCCACT	
1210	Cytochrome P450 (CytP450)	F	CCAGGACACGGATAGACTCG	52
		R	GAGTGGATACCGTGCTGACA	

4.4. Gene Expressions for Development Stages of Thalli and Cystocarp Maturation

To determine the transcript levels of two annotated *carbohydrate sulfotransferase* (henceforth *sulfotransferase*, *ST1* and *ST2*), and two *galactose-6 sulfurylase* (henceforth *sulfurylase*, *SY1* and *SY2*) genes, thalli of 100 mg each at different development stages (fertilised, fertile and infertile thalli) were frozen in liquid nitrogen and stored at −80 °C until the RNA was isolated.

To test if gene expression was affected by cystocarp maturity, levels of transcript expression were measured in accordance with the differentiation and development of the cystocarps in the apex of the thalli. In other words, well-developed cystocarps, and mature cystocarps—henceforth, fully-developed cystocarps. The presence of cystocarps was always reported during the spring (April). Pooled thalli containing cystocarps at different stages of development were used as a control. Infertile thalli were also used as a control for total absence of cystocarps (winter period, December).

4.5. Gene Expression Encoding Stress Proteins for Cystocarp Maturity

Levels of transcripts of two genes encoding stress proteins—i.e., *Cytochrome P450* (*Cyt P450*) and *WD40*—were determined by cystocarp maturity (well-developed and fully-developed cystocarps). The expressions of infertile thalli without cystocarps were used as controls.

4.6. Data Analysis

A one-way ANOVA followed by post hoc tests (Tukey HSD and Dunnett T3) were used to detect significant differences in gene transcript expression levels ($p < 0.01$) during the reproductive stage of thalli, maturity of the cystocarps and under stress.

Author Contributions: P.G.-J. conceived, designed and wrote the manuscript. S.R.M. conducted the experiments. P.G.-J. and R.R.R. discussed the manuscript. All authors have read and agreed to the published version of the manuscript.

Funding: This research was partially supported by the co-operation of the Ministry of Science, Innovation and University and of the University of Las Palmas de Gran Canaria. (Grant CGL2016-78442-C2-2-R, GOBESP2017-04 ULPGC and PROID2017010043 ACIISI; CEI2018-20 ULPGC) to P.G.J.

Conflicts of Interest: No conflicts of interest are declared.

References

1. Rees, D.A. Structure, conformation, and mechanism in the formation of polysaccharide gels and networks. *Adv. Carbohydr. Chem. Biochem.* **1969**, *24*, 267–332. [PubMed]
2. Murano, E.; Jellúš, V.; Piras, A.; Toffanin, R. Cell wall polysaccharides from Gelidium species: Physico-chemical studies using MRI techniques. *J. App. Phycol.* **1998**, *10*, 315–322. [CrossRef]
3. Usov, A.I. Polysaccharides of the red algae. In *Advance Carbohydrate Chemistry Biochemistry*; Horton, D., Ed.; Academic Press: Burlington, NJ, USA, 2011; Volume 65, pp. 115–217.
4. Tasende, M.G.; Cid, M.; Fraga, M.I. Qualitative and quantitative analysis of carrageenan content in gametophytes of Mastocarpus stellatus (Stackhouse) Guiry along Galician coast (NW Spain). *J. App. Phycol.* **2013**, *25*, 587–596. [CrossRef]
5. Van De Velde, F. Structure and function of hybrid carrageenans. *Food Hydrocoll.* **2008**, *22*, 727–734. [CrossRef]
6. Carrington, E.; Grace, S.P.; Chopin, T. Life history phases and the biomechanical properties of the red alga Chondrus crispus (Rhodophyta). *J. Phycol.* **2001**, *37*, 699–704. [CrossRef]
7. Garcia-Jimenez, P. Aclimatación Reproductiva, Fisiológica y Estructural al Cultivo In Vitro del Alga Grateloupia Doryphora (Montagne) Howe (Rhodophyta). Ph.D. Thesis, Universidad de Las Palmas de Gran Canaria, Las Palmas, Spain, 1994.
8. Garcia-Jimenez, P.; Robaina, R.R. Insight into the mechanism of red alga reproduction. What else is beyond cystocarps development? In *Systems Biology*; IntechOpen: London, UK, 2019. [CrossRef]
9. Garcia-Jimenez, P.; Montero-Fernández, M.; Robaina, R.R. Analysis of ethylene-induced gene regulation during carposporogenesis in the red seaweed Grateloupia imbricata (Rhodophyta). *J. Phycol.* **2018**, *54*, 681–689. [CrossRef]
10. Garcia-Jimenez, P.; Montero-Fernández, M.; Robaina, R.R. Molecular mechanisms underlying Grateloupia imbricata (Rhodophyta) carposporogenesis induced by methyl jasmonate. *J. Phycol.* **2017**, *53*, 1340–1344. [CrossRef]
11. Mittler, R. ROS are good. *Trends Plant Sci.* **2017**, *22*, 11–19. [CrossRef]
12. Tripathy, B.C.; Oelmüller, R. Reactive oxygen species generation and signalling in plants. *Plant Signal. Behav.* **2012**, *7*, 1621–1633. [CrossRef]
13. Xu, C.; Min, J. Structure and function of WD 40 domain proteins. *Protein Cell* **2011**, *2*, 202–214. [CrossRef]
14. Sun, T.; Tao, H.; Xie, J.; Zhang, S.; Xu, X. Degradation and antioxidant activity of k-carrageenans. *J. Appl. Polym. Sci.* **2010**, *117*, 194–199. [CrossRef]

15. Shukla, P.S.; Borza, T.; Critchley, A.T.; Prithiviraj, B. Carrageenans from red seaweeds as promoters of growth and elicitors of defense response in plants. *Front. Mar. Sci.* **2016**, *3*, 81. [CrossRef]
16. Genicot, S.; Préchoux, A.; Correc, G.; Kervarec, N.; Simon, G.; Craigie, J.S. Carrageenans: New tools for new applications. In *Blue Biotechnology: Production and Use of Marine Molecules*; La Barre, S., Bates, S.S., Eds.; Wiley-VCH Verlag GmbH & Co. KGaA: Weinheim, Germany, 2018; Volume 1, pp. 371–416. [CrossRef]
17. Genicot-Joncour, S.; Poinas, A.; Richard, O.; Potin, P.; Rudolph, B.; Kloareg, B.; Helbert, W. The cyclization of the 3, 6-anhydro-galactose ring of ι-carrageenan is catalyzed by two D-galactose-2, 6-sulfurylases in the red alga Chondrus crispus. *Plant Physiol.* **2009**, *151*, 1609–1616. [CrossRef] [PubMed]
18. Garcia-Jimenez, P.; Llorens, C.; Roig, F.J.; Robaina, R.R. Analysis of the transcriptome of the red seaweed Grateloupia imbricata with emphasis on reproductive potential. *Mar. Drugs* **2018**, *16*, 490. [CrossRef] [PubMed]
19. Popper, Z.A.; Tuohy, M.G. Beyond the green: Understanding the evolutionary puzzle of plant and algal cell walls. *Plant Physiol.* **2010**, *153*, 373–383. [CrossRef]
20. Torres, M.D.; Flórez-Fernández, N.; Domínguez, H. Integral utilization of red seaweed for bioactive production. *Mar. Drugs* **2019**, *17*, 314. [CrossRef]
21. Patel, S. Therapeutic importance of sulfated polysaccharides from seaweeds: Updating the recent findings. *Biotechnology* **2012**, *2*, 171–185. [CrossRef]
22. Cunha, L.; Grenha, A. Sulfated seaweed polysaccharides as multifunctional materials in drug delivery applications. *Mar. Drugs* **2016**, *14*, 42. [CrossRef]
23. Therkelsen, G.H. Carrageenan. In *Industrial Gums*; Academic Press: Cambridge, MA, USA, 1993; pp. 145–180.
24. Qin, X.; Ma, C.; Lou, Z.; Wang, A.; Wang, H. Purification and characterization of d-Gal-6-sulfurylase from Eucheuma striatum. *Carbohydr. Polym.* **2013**, *96*, 9–14. [CrossRef]
25. Lai, V.M.F.; Wong, P.A.-L.; Lii, C.-Y. Effects of cation properties on sol-gel transition and gel properties of κ-carrageenan. *J. Food Sci.* **2000**, *65*, 1332–1337. [CrossRef]
26. Casamassimi, A.; Ciccodicola, A. Transcriptional regulation: Molecules, involved mechanisms, and misregulation. *Int. J. Mol. Sci. Mar.* **2019**, *20*, 1281. [CrossRef] [PubMed]
27. Garcia-Jimenez, P.; Robaina, R.R. On reproduction in red algae: Further research needed at the molecular level. *Front. Plant Sci.* **2015**, *6*, 93. [PubMed]
28. Sacramento, A.T.; Garcia-Jimenez, P.; Robaina, R.R. The polyamine spermine induces cystocarp development in the seaweed Grateloupia (Rhodophyta). *Plant Growth Reg.* **2007**, *53*, 147–154. [CrossRef]
29. Hu, R.; Xiao, J.; Gu, T.; Yu, X.; Zhang, Y.; Chang, J.; He, G. Genome-wide identification and analysis of WD40 proteins in wheat (Triticum aestivum L.). *BMC Genom.* **2018**, *19*, 803.
30. Garcia-Jimenez, P.; Robaina, R.R. Effects of ethylene on tetrasporogenesis in Pterocladiella capillacea (Rhodophyta). *J. Phycol.* **2012**, *48*, 710–715. [CrossRef]
31. Vandesompele, J.; De Preter, K.; Pattyn, F.; Poppe, B.; Van Roy, N.; De Paepe, A.; Speleman, F. Accurate normalization of real-time quantitative RT-PCR data by geometric averaging of multiple internal control genes. *Genome Biol.* **2002**, *3*, research0034. [CrossRef]
32. Garcia-Jimenez, P.; García-Maroto, F.; Garrido-Cárdenas, J.A.; Ferrandiz, C.; Robaina, R.R. Differential expression of the ornithine decarboxylase gene during carposporogenesis in the thallus of the red seaweed Grateloupia imbricata (Halymeniaceae). *J. Plant Physiol.* **2009**, *166*, 1745-1754. [CrossRef]

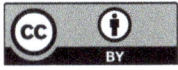

© 2020 by the authors. Licensee MDPI, Basel, Switzerland. This article is an open access article distributed under the terms and conditions of the Creative Commons Attribution (CC BY) license (http://creativecommons.org/licenses/by/4.0/).

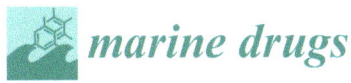

Article

Litoralimycins A and B, New Cytotoxic Thiopeptides from *Streptomonospora* sp. M2

Shadi Khodamoradi [1,2], Marc Stadler [2,3], Joachim Wink [1,2,*] and Frank Surup [2,3,*]

1. Microbial Strain Collection, Helmholtz-Centre for Infection Research (HZI), Inhoffenstr. 7, 38124 Braunschweig, Germany; shadi.khodamoradi@helmholtz-hzi.de
2. German Centre for Infection Research (DZIF), partner site Hannover-Braunschweig, 38124 Braunschweig, Germany; marc.stadler@helmholtz-hzi.de
3. Microbial Drugs Department, Helmholtz-Centre for Infection Research (HZI), Inhoffenstr. 7, 38124 Braunschweig, Germany
* Correspondence: joachim.wink@helmholtz-hzi.de (J.W.); frank.surup@helmholtz-hzi.de (F.S.); Tel.: +49-351-6181-4223 (J.W.); +49-351-6181-4256 (F.S.)

Received: 28 April 2020; Accepted: 20 May 2020; Published: 26 May 2020

Abstract: *Streptomonospora* sp. M2 has been isolated from a soil sample collected at the Wadden Sea beach in our ongoing program aimed at the isolation of rare Actinobacteria, ultimately targeting the discovery of new antibiotics. Because crude extracts derived from cultures of this strain showed inhibitory activity against the indicator organism *Bacillus subtilis*, it was selected for further analysis. HPLC–MS analysis of its culture broth revealed the presence of lipophilic metabolites. The two major metabolites of those were isolated by preparative reversed-phase HPLC and preparative TLC. Their planar structures were elucidated using high-resolution electrospray ionization mass spectrometry (HRESIMS), 1D and 2D NMR data as new thiopeptide antibiotics and named litoralimycin A (**1**) and B (**2**). Although rotating frame nuclear Overhauser effect spectroscopy (ROESY) data established a Z configuration of the $\Delta^{21,26}$ double bond, the stereochemistry of C-5 and C-15 were assigned as S by Marfey's method after ozonolysis. The biological activity spectrum of **1** and **2** is highly uncommon for thiopeptide antibiotics, since they showed only insignificant antibacterial activity, but **1** showed strong cytotoxic effects.

Keywords: thiopeptide antibiotic; screening; structure elucidation; natural products; rare actinobacteria

1. Introduction

New antibiotics in general and new types of antibiotics in particular are urgently needed to counter the increasing number of pathogenic bacteria resistant against present antibiotics [1]. Traditionally, actinobacteria have been the most prolific sources of novel antibiotics scaffolds, because many of the most important antimicrobials, such as β-lactames, tetracyclines, rifamycins, aminoglycosides, macrolides and glycopeptides, were discovered from them [2]. However, high rates of rediscovery of known compounds are observed when screening traditional producers, and the discovery of new molecules is getting more and more challenging. Therefore, current screening programs concentrate on discovering and isolating rare genera of microorganisms. Rare actinobacteria are regarded as actinomycete strains whose isolation frequency is much lower than that of *Streptomyces* spp. isolated by conventional methods. These rare actinobacteria are assessed as a potential storehouse for novel antibiotics due to their unique potential to produce novel metabolites [3,4].

The approach of utilizing rare organisms is accompanied by the screening of organisms from underexplored environments. Rare actinomycetes are widely distributed in terrestrial and aquatic ecosystems and the number of isolated genera and species is quickly increasing due to recently developed taxonomically selective isolation procedures, cultivation methods and genetic techniques [5]. We isolated the new strain *Streptomonospora* sp. M2 from a Wadden Sea sample collected at a beach near Cuxhaven, Germany, which is an underexplored environment. Since crude extracts of *Streptomonospora* sp. M2 showed inhibitory activity against Gram-positive indicator organisms including *Micrococcus luteus*, *Staphylococcus aureus* and *Bacillus subtilis*, the strain was selected for a detailed analysis of its bioactive secondary metabolites, yielding the isolation and structure elucidation of two new thiopeptide antibiotics (Figure 1) with an uncommon activity profile.

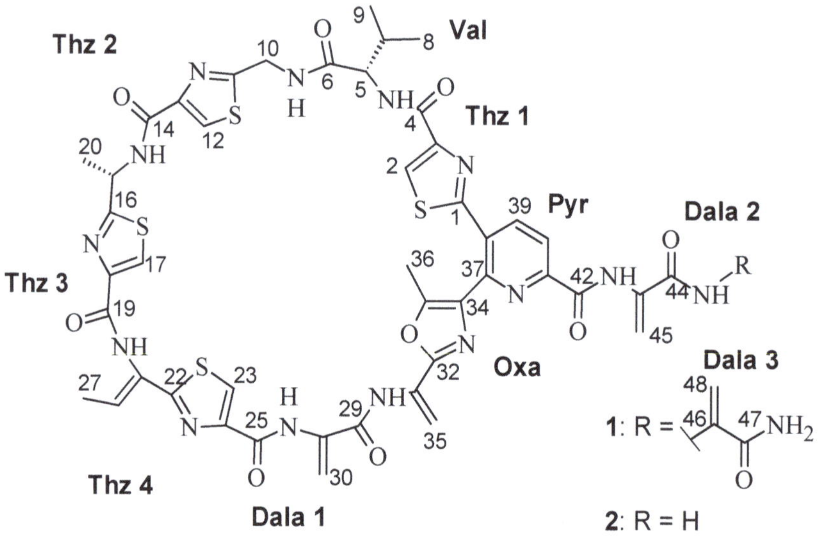

Figure 1. Chemical structure of **1** and **2**.

2. Results

2.1. Screening

By a fractionation of the crude extracts in 96-well plates, it was possible to link the antibacterial activity to a region containing two major peaks (Figure S1). Consequently, we isolated **1** and **2** by preparative HPLC.

2.2. Structure Elucidation

Litoralimycin A (**1**) was isolated as a light-yellow oil. The molecular formula of $C_{48}H_{45}N_{15}O_{10}S_4$ was derived from its high-resolution electrospray ionization mass spectrometry (HRESIMS) peak observed at *m/z* 1120.2429. ^{1}H and heteronuclear single-quantum correlation spectroscopy (HSQC) NMR spectra indicated the presence of 5 methyls, 4 exomethylenes and 1 low-field aliphatic methylene, and 7 olefinic/aromatic as well as 3 aliphatic methines, in addition to 10 exchangeable protons bound to heteroatoms (Table 1). The number of exomethylenes in combination with the four sulfur atoms gave an early hint towards a thiopeptide. The ^{13}C spectrum indicated the presence of 9 additional carbonyls as well as 19 further olefinic carbons bearing no hydrogens. Based on correlation spectroscopy (COSY), total correlation spectroscopy (TOCSY) and heteronuclear multiple-bond correlation spectroscopy (HMBC) correlations, the planar thiopeptide structure, containing four thiazole (Thz), a valine (Val), an oxazole (Oxa), a pyridine (Pyr) and three dehydroalanine (Dala) units, was established (Figure 2). The rotating frame nuclear Overhauser effect spectroscopy (ROESY) correlation between H$_3$-27 and 21-NH established the $\Delta^{21,26}$ double bond geometry as *Z*. Since thiazole amino acids racemize very easily during acid hydrolosis, the configuration of C-15 was determined by ozonolysis of the aromatic ring for preservation of the chiral center followed by acid hydrolosis [6]. After ozonolysis, hydrolyzation and derivatization with FDAA, we detected L-Val and L-Ala according to Marfey's method [7]. Thus, both C-5 and C-15 are S-configured.

Table 1. NMR data (^{1}H 700 MHz, ^{13}C 175 MHZ) of 1 in DMSO-d_6.

Unit	Pos	δ_C	δ_H	Unit	Pos	δ_C	δ_H
Thz 1	1	163.6, C		Dala 1	28	133.7, C	
	2	127.1, CH	8.47, s		28NH	NH	9.70, br s
	3	149.3, C			29	162.5, C	
	4	159.9, C			30	104.5, CH$_2$	5.74, br s
Val	5	58.2, CH	4.38, dd (9.3, 7.4)		30		6.49, br s
	5NH	NH	8.08, d (9.3)	Oxa	31	129.0, C	
	6	170.9, C			31NH	NH	9.78, br s
	5	30.6, CH	2.11, m		32	155.8, C	
	8	19.3, CH$_3$	0.91, d (6.7)		33	150.0, C	
	9	18.4, CH$_3$	0.88, d (6.7)		34	133.1, C	
Thz 2	10	40.2, CH$_2$	4.55, m		35	109.5, CH$_2$	5.64, br s
			4.70, dd (16.0, 6.4)				5.43, br s
	10NH	NH	8.95, t (6.4)		36	11.4, CH$_3$	2.60, s
	11	168.6, C		Pyr	37	147.6, C	
	12	125.3, CH	8.25, s		38	130.8, C	
	13	148.6, C			39	141.1, CH	8.60, d (8.1)
	14	159.9, C			40	121.1, CH	8.25, d (8.1)
Thz 3	15	46.8, CH	5.44, m		41	149.0, C	
	15NH	NH	8.74, d (8.2)		42	161.4, C	
	16	173.5, C		Dala 2	43	134.0, C	
	17	125.1, CH	8.29, m		43NH	NH	10.5, br s
	18	148.7, C			44	161.9, C	
	19	159.2, C			45	104.0, CH$_2$	5.82, br s
	20	20.5, CH$_3$	1.55, d (6.9)				6.61, br s
Thz 4	21	129.2, C		Dala 3	46	135.3, C	
	21NH	NH	9.80, br s		46NH	NH	9.54, br s
	22	167.3, C			47	165.1, C	
	23	125.0, CH	8.31, s		47NH	NH$_2$	7.48, br s
	24	148.5, C				NH$_2$	7.91, br s
	25	158.8, C			48	106.7, CH$_2$	5.96, s
	26	128.3, CH	6.52, d (6.9)				5.67, s
	27	14.1, CH$_3$	1.79, d (6.9)				

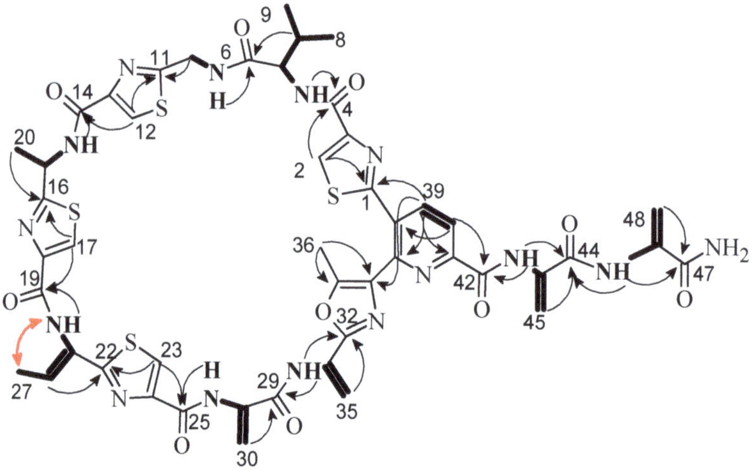

Figure 2. Selected ^{1}H,^{1}H COSY (bold lines), ^{1}H,^{13}C HMBC (black arrows) and ^{1}H,^{1}H NOESY (red arrow) correlations of **1**.

HRESIMS data of **2** gave a molecular formula of $C_{45}H_{42}N_{14}O_9S_4$, implying the formal loss of a C_3H_3NO fragment compared to **1**. The proton and carbon NMR spectra of **2** were highly similar to those of **1**, with the key difference of the absence of a terminal dehydroalanin moiety. Therefore, the structure of **2** was established as identical to that of **1** with its side chain truncated by one dehydroalanin moiety.

2.3. Bioactivity

Litoralimycins A (**1**) and B (**2**) were evaluated for their minimum inhibitory concentration (MIC). Both compounds showed only a very weak activity against *Staphylococcus aureus* Newman and *Bacillus subtilis* DSM10^T with MIC values of 66.7 µg/mL, respectively. No further effects were detected against any Gram-negative bacteria or fungi. (Table S1). However, cytotoxic effects against different cell lines were detected for **1** (Table 2). Litoralimycin B (**2**) with its truncated side chain showed much weaker cytotoxic activity.

Table 2. Cytotoxic activities of litoralimycins A (**1**) and B (**2**) against different cell lines. Values indicate IC$_{50}$ in µg/mL.

Compound	L929	KB3.1	MCF-7	SKOV-3	A431	PC-3
1	2.9	2.6	1.0	28	0.8	31
2	24.0	/	n.t. ^{1}	n.t.	n.t	n.t
epothilon B [8]	0.00082	0.000065	0.000048	0.000095	0.000045	0.0001

^{1} n.t.: not tested

3. Discussion

Thiopeptides, or thiazolyl peptides, are highly modified sulfur-rich peptides of ribosomal origin. Over 100 chemical entities have been isolated in the last 50 years [9]. Of these entities, thiostrepton has been used as an FDA-approved active pharmaceutical ingredient for animals, and nosiheptide has been widely applied in veterinary antibiotics and food preservation. Their most characteristic feature is the central nitrogen-containing six-membered ring structure. Depending on the oxidation state of this central ring, thiopeptides can be classified into five different series [10]. The litoralimycins belong to the *d* series, which is the most numerous subgroup, due to their trisubstituted pyridine moiety.

Another option to group the thiopeptides is based on the ring size of the main macrocycle, since ring sizes of 26, 29, 32 and 35 atoms are found. Specifically, litoralimycins **1** and **2** belong to a small family of compounds with an oxazolyl-thiazolyl-pyridine fragment embedded in a 35-membered (13-residue) peptidyl macrocycle [11]. Other members of this family, which have highest structural similarity to **1** and **2**, are the berninamycins, sulfomycin, thioplabin and TP-1161A. Common variations between members of this family are the exchange of thiazole by oxazole moieties, different methylation patterns and the size of the side chain (see Figure S3).

Most characterized thiopeptides display nanomolar potency toward Gram-positive bacteria by blocking protein translation, including the notorious pathogens methicillin-resistant *Staphylococcus aureus* (MRSA), vancomycin-resistant enterococci (VRE), and penicillin-resistant *Streptococcus pneumoniae* (PRSP). Their mechanism of action, acting as protein synthesis inhibitors, correlates with the size of the primary macrocycle: 29-atom macrocycles bind to elongation factor EF-TU, while 26- and 32-atom macrocycles bind to the interface of protein L11 and the 23S rRNA within the 50S ribosomal subunit. The general molecular target of compounds with the largest 35-membered macrocycle remains unknown [10], although berninamycin was reported to target the 50S ribosome, in a similar manner to thiostrepton [11].

Using NMR and biochemical assays, a three-dimensional interaction model was developed, identifying L-Thr as a preserved region for the interaction with the ribosome/L11 complex [12]. This residue is missing for the litoralimycins, since **1** and **2** bear a L-Val at this position instead. In conformity with **1** and **2**, radamycin also has a mutated residue with L-Val replacing L-Thr. In analogy to the litoralimycins, radamycin was devoid of any antibacterial activity in agar diffusion assays [13,14]. Nevertheless, radamycin showed a strong *tipA* promoting activity. *tipA* gene promotion, encoding the two thiostrepton-induced proteins (Tip) TipAL and TipAS. The latter serves as a defense mechanism for bacteria against thiopeptides. Since the *tipA* promotion activity was identified to be dependent on a dehydroalanine-containing tail close to the six-membered central scaffold [15], we expect the litoralimycins to be *tipA* activators.

Besides the aforementioned effects on bacteria, some thiopeptides show good anticancer activities [9]. For thiostrepton it was shown that this activity is based on its effect of reducing transcriptional activity of the forkhead box M1 (FOXM1). FOXM1 is an oncogenic transcription factor that is upregulated in a wide range of cancers. It is involved in the regulation of the cell cycle and promotes angiogenesis, as well as metastasis. Because treatment with thiostrepton had an effect on cell proliferation and cell-cycle progression in MCF-7 cells [16], and litoralimycins A (**1**) was strongly active against cell line MCF-7 in our test assay, FOXM1 might be the molecular target in common.

4. Materials and Methods

4.1. General

HRESIMS mass spectra were measured with an Agilent 1200 series HPLC–UV system in combination with an ESI-TOF-MS (Maxis, Bruker) (column 2.1 × 50 mm, 1.7 µm, C18 Acquity UPLC BEH (Waters), solvent A: H_2O + 0.1% formic acid, solvent B: ACN + 0.1% formic acid, gradient: 5% B for 0.5 min increasing to 100% B in 19.5 min, maintaining 100% B for another 5 min, RF = 0.6 mL min^{-1}, UV detection 200–600 nm). NMR spectra were recorded on a Bruker Avance III 700 MHz spectrometer with a 5 mm TCI cryoprobe (^{1}H 700 MHz, ^{13}C 175 MHz, ^{15}N 71 MHz). Chemical shifts δ were referenced to DMSO-d_6 (^{1}H, δ = 2.50 ppm; ^{13}C, δ = 39.51 ppm). UV spectra were recorded using the Shimadzu UV*vis* spectrophotometer UV-2450. Optical rotation was determined using a PerkinElmer 241 polarimeter. Preparative isolation of the major components was achieved with preparative HPLC-system Gilson PLc 2250 (C18 column-nucleodur-7 µm-125 × 40 mm-RP 100, using Solvent A: H_2O, solvent B: acetonitrile, gradient system: 20% B for 0.5 min increasing to 50% B in 30 min, 50% B to 100% B for 20 min, maintaining 100% B for 5 min, flow rate = 50 mL/min, detection at 200–600 nm).

4.2. Strain Maintenance

Streptomonospora sp. DSM 106425T was isolated in 2017 by the serial dilution method from a sand sample that had been collected from a beach of the North Sea at Cuxhaven, Germany. The strain grew well in the presence of 7% NaCl. This percentage of sodium chloride was added to all media that we used for culturing and production media. A section of the agar containing bacterial colonies and aerial mycelium was stored in glycerol 20% at −80 °C. The strain was transferred to 100 mL of liquid GYM medium (0.4% glucose, 0.4% yeast extract, 1% malt extract, 0.2% $CaCO_3$; pH 7.2). The inoculated flask was incubated on a rotary shaker (160 rpm) for 5 days at 30 °C.

4.3. Fermentation, Extraction, and Isolation of Compounds

The 5-day-old preculture was transferred to production medium 1:10 in eight 1000-mL flasks, filled with 800 mL of medium 5294 (1% soluble starch, 0.2% yeast extract, 1% glucose, 1% glycerol, 0.25% corn steep liquor, 0.2% peptone, 0.1% NaCl, 0.3% $CaCO_3$; pH 7.2) incubated at 30 °C for 8 days on rotary shaker (160 rpm). The 8-day-old culture medium was centrifuged using a Sorvall RC-5 refrigerated superspeed centrifuge for 30 min, at 8500 rpm. The supernatant was discarded and 311 g cell mass was extracted with two liters of acetone three time in an ultrasonic bath (3 × 30 min). The solution obtained was evaporated to yield an aqueous phase, which was further extracted with ethyl acetate (3 × 500 mL) and the ethyl acetate portion was dried out with evaporator to yield 575.2 mg of crude cell mass extract. An initial pre-separation of 575.2 mg crude extract was applied with a Strata TM-X 33 UM Polymeric reversed phase 1 g/12 mL Giga tube (Phenomenex) and washed three times with methanol. Subsequently, fractionation of 265.2 mg crude extract was completed by preparative HPLC (Gilson) (1 run using a linear gradient of solvent B from 20% to 50% solvent B in 30 min, 50% to 100% B in 20 min followed by isocratic conditions for 10 min at a flow rate of 50 mL/min). Fractions were collected and combined according to UV absorption at 220, 280 and 350 nm and yielded 5.6 mg of **1** at a retention time of 37.5–38.5 min and 0.5 mg of **2** at 36.5–37 min, respectively.

Litoralimycin A (**1**): light-yellow oil; $[\alpha]_D$ = +251 (*c* = 1 mg/mL in acetone); ^{1}H NMR (700 MHz, DMSO-d_6): see Table 1; ^{13}C NMR (175 MHz, DMSO-d_6): see Table 1; ESI-MS: *m/z* 1120.38 [M + H]$^+$, 1118.43 [M + H]$^+$; HRESIMS: *m/z* 1120.2429 [M + H]$^+$ (calcd. for $C_{48}H_{46}N_{15}O_{10}S_4$ 1120.2429), 1142.2246 [M + Na]$^+$ (calcd. for $C_{48}H_{45}N_{15}O_{10}S_4Na$ 1142.2249).

Litoralimycin B (**2**): light-yellow oil; $[\alpha]_D$ = +399 (*c* = 1 mg/mL in acetone); ^{1}H NMR (700 MHz, DMSO-d_6): δ_H 10.67 (br s, 43–NH), 9.81 (br s, 21–NH), 9.74 (br s, 31–NH), 9.69 (br s, 28–NH), 8.95 (dd, *J* = 6.2, 5.2 Hz, 10–NH), 8.75 (br d, *J* = 8.2 Hz, 15–NH), 8.52 (d, *J* = 8.2 Hz, 39–H), 8.45 (s, 2–H), 8.31 (s, 23–H), 8.29 (s, 17–H), 8.25 (s, 12–H), 8.22 (d, *J* = 8.2 Hz, 40–H), 8.17 (br s, 44–NH$_a$), 8.07 (br d, *J* = 9.2 Hz, 5–NH), 7.66 (br s, 44–NH$_b$), 6.58 (s, 45–H$_a$), 6.52 (q, *J* = 6.9 Hz, 26–H), 6.48 (br s, 30–H$_a$), 5.81 (br s, 45–H$_b$), 5.72 (br s, 30–H$_b$), 5.63 (br s, 35–H$_a$), 5.44 (m, 15–H), 5.42 (br s, 35–H$_b$), 4.70 (dd, *J* = 15.9, 6.2 Hz, 10–H$_a$), 4.54 (dd, *J* = 15.9, 5.2 Hz, 10–H$_b$), 4.37 (dd, *J* = 9.2, 7.3 Hz, 5–H), 2.64 (s, 36–H$_3$), 2.10 (dspt, *J* = 7.2, 6.9 Hz, 7–H), 1.79 (br d, *J* = 6.9 Hz, 27–H$_3$), 1.55 (br d, *J* = 6.9 Hz, 20–H$_3$), 0.90 (d, *J* = 6.9 Hz, 9–H$_3$), 0.87 (d, *J* = 6.9 Hz, 8–H$_3$) ppm; ^{13}C NMR (175 MHz, DMSO-d_6): δ_C 173.6 (C, C–16), 170.9 (C, C–6), 168.6 (C, C–11), 167.3 (C, C–22), 164.9 (C, C–44), 163.8 (C, C–1), 161.2 (C, C–42), 159.98 (C, C–4), 159.94 (C, C–14), 159.2 (C, C–19), 158.9 (C, C–25), 155.6 (C, C–32), 150.2 (C, C–33), 149.22 (C, C–3), 149.18 (C, C–41), 148.7 (C, C–18), 148.6 (2xC, C–13, C–24), 147.7 (C, C–37), 141.2 (CH, C–39), 133.8 (C, C–28), 133.6 (C, C–43), 133.1 (C, C–34), 130.6 (C, C–38), 129.2 (C, C–21), 129.0 (C, C–31), 128.3 (CH, C–26), 125.3 (CH, C–12), 125.1 (CH, C–17), 125.0 (CH, C–23), 104.5 (CH$_2$, C–30), 102.5 (CH$_2$, C–45), 58.2 (CH, C–5), 46.9 (CH, C–15), 40.0 (CH$_2$, C–10), 30.7 (CH, C–7), 20.6 (CH$_3$, C–20), 19.3 (CH$_3$, C–8), 18.4 (CH$_3$, C–9), 14.2 (CH$_3$, C–27), 11.6 (CH$_3$, C–26); ESI-MS: *m/z* 1051.32 [M + H]$^+$, 1049.34 [M + H]$^+$; HRESIMS: *m/z* 1051.2219 [M + H]$^+$ (calcd. for $C_{45}H_{43}N_{14}O_9S_4$ 1051.2215), 1073.2031 [M + Na]$^+$ (calcd. for $C_{45}H_{42}N_{14}O_9S_4Na$ 1073.2034).

4.4. Ozonolysis, Hydrolysis and Marfey's Derivatization with L-FDAA

For the ozonolysis reaction a stream of O_3 was bubbled through a solution of **1** (2.3 mg) dissolved in methanol (6 mL) at −78 °C until the solution obtained a characteristic blue color and stirred for 30 min. Subsequently, the solvent was removed in vacuo and the resulting oxidized material was subjected to hydrolysis in 3 mL of 6 N HCl at 110 °C for 24 h as described in [6]. Afterwards, the solvent was removed under a stream of nitrogen for 3 h and the remainder dissolved in H_2O (200 µL), of which 100 µL were proceeded further. A total of 1 N $NaHCO_3$ (20 µL) and 1% 1-fluoro-2,4-dinitrophenyl-5-Lalaninamide (100 µL in acetone) were added, and the mixture was heated at 40 °C for 40 min [17]. After being cooled to room temperature, the solutions were neutralized with 2 N HCl (20 µL) and evaporated to dryness. The residues were dissolved in MeOH and analyzed by HPLC–MS. Retention times in minutes of FDAA-derivatized amino acids were 6.5 for Val and 5.0 for Ala. Retention times of the authentic amino acid standards were L-Val 6.5, DL-Val 6.5/7.5, L-Ala 5.0, DL-Ala 5.0/6.0.

4.5. Minimum Inhibitory Concentrations

Minimum Inhibitory Concentrations (MIC) were investigated in a serial dilution assay in 96-well microtiter plates in YM medium for yeasts and filamentous fungi and BD™ Difco™ Müller-Hinton Broth for bacteria, as previously published [18].

4.6. Cytotoxicity Assay

The in vitro cytotoxicity assay was carried out as described earlier [8].

4.7. HPLC Fractionation and Bioassays in 96-Well Plates

An Agilent 1260 Series HPLC–UV system equipped with a Waters, XBridge BEHC18, 2.1 mm 100 mm column (pore size 135 Å, particle size 3.5 µm, solvent A: H_2O-acetonitrile (95/5), 5 mmol NH_4Ac, 0.04 mL/L CH_3COOH; solvent B: H_2O-acetonitrile (5/95), 5 mmol NH_4Ac, 0.04 mL/L CH_3COOH; gradient system: 10% B increasing to 100% B in 30 min; flow rate 0.3 mL/min; 40 °C; UV-detection at 210–450 nm) was used for the chromatographic fractionation of crude extracts. The same HPLC gradient was used as for the high-resolution electrospray ionization mass spectrometry (HRESIMS) instrument. The flow-through was collected in 30 s intervals into a 96-well microtiter plate. Afterwards, the plates were dried by a constant nitrogen-flush for 40 min, inoculated with 150 mL indicator bacteria per well and incubated as described [17]. After 24 h the plates were evaluated and documented employing a custom-made mirror stand and a CANON EOS 60D digital camera.

5. Conclusions

Two new thiopeptide antibiotics were isolated from a new actinomycetes bacterium, which was isolated from a sand sample collected at a Wadden Sea beach. While their planar structures were elucidated by NMR and MS data, their absolute configuration was determined by degradation by ozonolysis and hydrolosis followed by Marfey's method. Their spectrum of biological activities is rare, because they are cytotoxic but possess virtually no antibacterial activities.

Supplementary Materials: The following are available online at http://www.mdpi.com/1660-3397/18/6/280/s1, Figure S1: Fractionation analysis of *Streptomonospora* sp. M2 crude extract. Table S1: Antimicrobial activity of **1** and **2**, Figure S2: Observed TOCSY, HMBC and ROESY correlations for **1**, Figure S3: Known compounds structurally related to litoralimycins, Figure S4: HPLC–MS and UV–Vis chromatograms of *Streptomonospora* sp. M2 and HRESIMS data, Figure S5: HPLC–ESIMS spectrum of litoralimycin A (**1**), Figure S6: ^{1}H NMR spectrum (700 MHz, DMSO-d_6) of litoralimycin A (**1**), Figure S7: ^{13}C NMR spectrum (175 MHz, DMSO-d_6) of litoralimycin A (**1**), Figure S8: COSY NMR spectrum (700 MHz, DMSO-d_6) of litoralimycin A (**1**), Figure S9: ROESY NMR spectrum (700 MHz, DMSO-d_6) of litoralimycin A (**1**), Figure S10: HSQC NMR spectrum (700 MHz, DMSO-d_6) of litoralimycin A (**1**), Figure S11: HMBC NMR spectrum (700 MHz, DMSO-d_6) of litoralimycin A (**1**), Figure S12: Marfey derivatization for determination of type and configuration of amino acids in litoralimycin A (**1**), Figure S13: HPLC-ESIMS spectrum of litoralimycin B (**2**), Figure S14: ^{1}H NMR spectrum (700 MHz, DMSO-d_6) of litoralimycin B (**2**), Figure S15: ^{13}C NMR spectrum (175 MHz, DMSO-d_6) of litoralimycin B (**2**), Figure S16:

COSY NMR spectrum (700 MHz, DMSO-d_6) of litoralimycin B (**2**), Figure S17: ROESY NMR spectrum (700 MHz, DMSO-d_6) of litoralimycin B (**2**), Figure S18: HSQC NMR spectrum (700 MHz, DMSO-d_6) of litoralimycin B (**2**), Figure S19: HMBC NMR spectrum (700 MHz, DMSO-d_6) of litoralimycin B (**2**), Figure S20: MS/MS data for **1** and **2** with fragmentation of $[M + Na]^+$ ions.

Author Contributions: Conceptualization, J.W. and F.S.; execution of experiments, S.K.; structure elucidation, F.S.; resources, M.S.; writing—original draft preparation, S.K.; writing—review and editing, M.S., J.W., F.S.; supervision, J.W., F.S.; funding acquisition, M.S., J.W. All authors have read and agreed to the published version of the manuscript.

Funding: This research was funded by a personal stipend to S.K.

Acknowledgments: We would also like to thank Klaus-Peter Conrad for the measurement of HRESIMS data, Wera Collisi for conducting the bioassays, and Christel Kakoschke for the measurement of NMR spectra. We gratefully acknowledge the assistance of Romy Schade in cultivation of the strain and Silke Reinecke for helping to isolate the metabolites.

Conflicts of Interest: The authors declare no conflict of interest.

References

1. Stadler, M.; Dersch, P. How to overcome the antibiotic crisis—Facts, challenges, technologies & future perspectives. *Curr. Top Microbiol. Immunol.* **2017**, *398*, 496.
2. Genilloud, O. Actinomycetes: Still a source of novel antibiotics. *Nat. Prod. Rep.* **2017**, *34*, 1203–1232. [CrossRef] [PubMed]
3. Tiwari, K.; Gupta, R.K. Rare actinomycetes: A potential storehouse for novel antibiotics. *Crit. Rev. Biotechnol.* **2012**, *32*, 108–132. [CrossRef] [PubMed]
4. Landwehr, W.; Wolf, C.; Wink, J. Actinobacteria and myxobacteria—Two of the most important bacterial resources for novel antibiotics. In *How to Overcome the Antibiotic Crisis*; Springer: Cham, Switzerland, 2016; pp. 273–302.
5. Subramani, R.; Aalbersberg, W. Culturable rare *Actinomycetes*: Diversity, isolation and marine natural product discovery. *Appl. Microbiol. Biotechnol.* **2013**, *97*, 9291–9321. [CrossRef] [PubMed]
6. Yun, B.-S.; Fujita, K.; Furihata, K.; Seto, H. Absolute stereochemistry and solution conformation of promothiocins. *Tetrahedron* **2001**, *57*, 9683–9687. [CrossRef]
7. Marfey, P.; Ottensen, M. Determination of D-amino acids. I. Hydrolysis of DNP-L-amino acid methyl esters with carboxypeptidase-Y. *Carlsberg Res. Commun.* **1984**, *49*, 585–590. [CrossRef]
8. Surup, F.; Halecker, S.; Nimtz, M.; Rodrigo, S.; Schulz, B.; Steinert, M.; Stadler, M. Hyfraxins A and B, cytotoxic ergostane-type steroid and lanostane triterpenoid glycosides from the invasive ash dieback ascomycete *Hymenoscyphus fraxineus*. *Steroids* **2018**, *135*, 92–97. [CrossRef] [PubMed]
9. Shen, X.; Mustafa, M.; Chen, Y.; Cao, Y.; Gao, J. Natural thiopeptides as a privileged scaffold for drug discovery and therapeutic development. *Med. Chem. Res.* **2019**, *28*, 1063–1098. [CrossRef]
10. Just-Baringo, X.; Albericio, F.; Álvarez, M. Thiopeptide antibiotics: Retrospective and recent advances. *Mar. Drugs* **2014**, *12*, 317–351. [CrossRef]
11. Malcolmson, S.J.; Young, T.S.; Ruby, J.G.; Skewes-Cox, P.; Walsh, C.T. The posttranslational modification cascade to the thiopeptide berninamycin generates linear forms and altered macrocyclic scaffolds. *Proc. Natl. Acad. Sci. USA* **2013**, *110*, 8483–8488. [CrossRef] [PubMed]
12. Lentzen, G.; Klinck, R.; Matassova, N.; Aboul-ela, F.; Murchie, A.I.H. Structural Basis for Contrasting Activities of Ribosome Binding Thiazole Antibiotics. *Chem. Biol.* **2003**, *10*, 769–778. [CrossRef]
13. González Holgado, G.; Castro Rodríguez, J.; Cañedo Hernández, L.M.; Díaz, M.; Fernández-Abalos, J.M.; Trujillano, I.; Santamaría, R.I. Radamycin, a novel thiopeptide produced by *Streptomyces* sp. RSP9. I. Taxonomy, fermentation, isolation and biological activities. *J. Antibiot.* **2002**, *55*, 383–390. [CrossRef] [PubMed]
14. Castro Rodríguez, J.; González Holgado, G.; Santamaría Sánchez, R.I.; Cañedo, L.M. Radamycin, a novel thiopeptide produced by *Streptomyces* sp. RSP9. II. Physico-chemical properties and structure determination. *J. Antibiot.* **2002**, *55*, 391–395. [CrossRef] [PubMed]
15. Chiu, M.L.; Folcher, M.; Katoh, T.; Puglia, A.M.; Vohradsky, J.; Yun, B.S.; Seto, H.; Thompson, C.J. Broad spectrum thiopeptide recognition specificity of the *Streptomyces lividans* TipAL protein and its role in regulating gene expression. *J. Biol. Chem.* **1999**, *274*, 20578–20586. [CrossRef] [PubMed]

16. Hegdem, N.S.; Sanders, D.A.; Rodriguez, R.; Balasubramanian, S. The transcription factor FOXM1 is a cellular target of the natural product thiostrepton. *Nat. Chem.* **2011**, *3*, 725–731. [CrossRef] [PubMed]
17. Viehrig, K.; Surup, F.; Harmrolfs, K.; Jansen, R.; Kunze, B.; Müller, R. Concerted action of P450 plus helper protein to form the amino-hydroxy-piperidone moiety of the potent protease inhibitor Crocapeptin. *J. Am. Chem. Soc.* **2013**, *135*, 16885–16894. [CrossRef] [PubMed]
18. Sandargo, B.; Michehl, M.; Praditya, D.; Steinmann, E.; Stadler, M.; Surup, F. Antiviral meroterpenoid rhodatin and sesquiterpenoids rhodocoranes A–E from the wrinkled peach mushroom, *Rhodotus palmatus*. *Org. Lett.* **2019**, *21*, 3286–3289. [CrossRef] [PubMed]

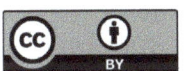

© 2020 by the authors. Licensee MDPI, Basel, Switzerland. This article is an open access article distributed under the terms and conditions of the Creative Commons Attribution (CC BY) license (http://creativecommons.org/licenses/by/4.0/).

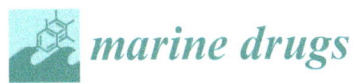

Article

Effects of Sulfated Fucans from *Laminaria hyperborea* Regarding VEGF Secretion, Cell Viability, and Oxidative Stress and Correlation with Molecular Weight

Philipp Dörschmann [1,*], Georg Kopplin [2,3], Johann Roider [1] and Alexa Klettner [1]

1. Department of Ophthalmology, University Medical Center, University of Kiel, Arnold-Heller-Str. 3, Haus 25, 24105 Kiel, Germany; Johann.Roider@uksh.de (J.R.); Alexa.Klettner@uksh.de (A.K.)
2. Alginor ASA, Haraldsgata 162, 5525 Haugesund, Norway; Georg@alginor.no
3. Norwegian Biopolymer Laboratory (NOBIPOL), Department of Biotechnology and Food Science, NTNU, 7491 Trondheim, Norway; Georg.Kopplin@ntnu.no
* Correspondence: philipp.doerschmann@uksh.de; Tel.: +49-431-500-13712

Received: 29 August 2019; Accepted: 23 September 2019; Published: 25 September 2019

Abstract: Background: Sulfated fucans show interesting effects in the treatment of ocular diseases (e.g., age-related macular degeneration), depending on their chemical structure. Here, we compared three purified sulfated fucans from *Laminaria hyperborea* (LH) regarding cell viability, oxidative stress protection, and vascular endothelial growth factor (VEGF) secretion in ocular cells. Methods: High-molecular-weight sulfated fucan (M_w = 1548.6 kDa, Fuc1) was extracted with warm water and purified through ultrafiltration. Lower-molecular-weight samples (M_w = 499 kDa, Fuc2; 26.9 kDa, Fuc3) were obtained by mild acid hydrolysis of ultrapurified sulfated fucan and analyzed (SEC-MALS (Size-exclusion chromatography-Multi-Angle Light Scattering), ICP-MS, and GC). Concentrations between 1 and 100 µg/mL were tested. Cell viability was measured after 24 h (uveal melanoma cell line (OMM-1), retinal pigment epithelium (RPE) cell line ARPE-19, primary RPE cells) via MTT/MTS (3-(4,5-dimethylthiazol-2-yl)-2,5-diphenyltetrazolium bromide/3-(4,5-Dimethylthiazol-2-yl)-5-(3-carboxymethoxyphenyl)-2-(4-sulfophenyl)-2H-tetrazolium) assay. Oxidative stress protection was determined after 24 h (OMM-1, ARPE-19). VEGF secretion was analyzed via ELISA after three days (ARPE-19, RPE). Results: Fuc2 and Fuc3 were antiproliferative for OMM-1, but not for ARPE. Fuc1 protected OMM-1. VEGF secretion was lowered with all fucans except Fuc3 in ARPE-19 and RPE. The results suggest a correlation between molecular weight and biological activity, with efficiency increasing with size. Conclusion: The LH sulfated fucan Fuc1 showed promising results regarding VEGF inhibition and protection, encouraging further medical research.

Keywords: fucoidan; fucan; age-related macular degeneration; VEGF; oxidative stress; *Laminaria hyperborea*; brown seaweed extracts; proliferation; molecular weight; retinal pigment epithelium

1. Introduction

Laminaria hyperborea (LH), commonly known as tangle or cuvie, belongs to the large brown seaweed family of the Laminariaceae (alias kelp). It mainly grows in the northeast Atlantic Ocean, especially around Scandinavia. LH, like all brown algal species, contains fucose-containing sulfated polysaccharides (FCSP), commonly known as fucoidan, as a cell wall component. FCSP predominantly based on sulfated L-fucose residues are defined as sulfated fucans [1]. FCSP are a very heterogeneous group of polysaccharides with strong variations in sugar composition, degree of branching and sulfation, and molecular weight. Their structure depends on different aspects, like species, harvest time, place, and extraction method [2]. This heterogeneity in structures also leads to a variety of different biological activities. Sulfated fucans have been described as being able to reduce oxidative stress and inflammation, as well as being capable of interfering with vascular endothelial growth factor (VEGF) and blood lipids [3]. These properties render sulfated fucans very interesting for medical purposes, especially for the treatment of age-related macular degeneration (AMD) [4]. AMD is the main cause of blindness in the industrialized world and may cause an irreversible loss in central vision in the elderly due to the degeneration of photoreceptors within the macula lutea. This may happen in two ways: starting in the early phase with the deposition of drusen and an accumulation of lipid peroxidation products (lipofuscin), it may progress to dry AMD, where retinal pigment epithelium (RPE) degeneration is followed by a death of photoreceptors, leading to geographical atrophy of the retina as a late stage [5,6]. In wet AMD, the major growth factor of blood vessels, VEGF, is abnormally increased, leading to the growth of blood vessels under and into the retina. Followed by edema and sometimes bleeding, it leads to a disruption of the retina [5]. The pathology of AMD is based on four molecular mechanisms that increase the risk of this illness: inflammation, complement activation, oxidative burden, and disturbed VEGF generation [5,7–9]. The only therapy possibility is repeated anti-VEGF injections into the eyes of the patient [10], which slows down the pathology of wet AMD.

Because of their biological activities, FCSP are very interesting as possible new therapeutics for the treatment of AMD [3]. We showed previously that commercial sulfated fucan from *Fucus vesiculosus* reduces VEGF and the angiogenesis of RPE cells [4]. We also described the protective effects of *Saccharina latissima* (SL) sulfated fucan for ARPE-19 cells against oxidative stress insult; this fucan also lowered VEGF in ARPE-19 and RPE cells [11]. Other extracts from *Fucus serratus*, *Fucus distichus* subsp. *evanescens*, and *Laminaria digitata* also inhibited VEGF secretion in ARPE-19 cells [11]. The chemical structure and composition of sulfated fucan from LH has been previously described [12]. It was shown that the biological activity of LH sulfated fucan is dependent on the molecular weight and the degree of sulfation [12]. LH sulfated fucans with higher molecular weight and degree of sulfation were capable to reduce coagulation and had anti-inflammatory effects [12]. Stefaniak-Vidarsson et al. (2017) described the anti-proliferative effects of *Laminaria* sulfated fucans in activated human macrophages and showed that these sulfated fucans triggered tumor necrosis factor-α and interleukins 6 and 10 [13]. However, only few reports about the activity of LH sulfated fucans can be found in the literature. Because of the described connected effects to molecular weight and to the high degree of sulfation, as well as the different species-dependent structures and activities, we tested LH sulfated fucans additionally to the other mentioned species to find the best sulfated fucans for further AMD-relevant research.

With this study we wanted to investigate whether these LH sulfated fucans display toxic effects and whether they are capable of interfering with VEGF secretion and the oxidative burden in ocular cells, with a view to making an important step further to new AMD treatment possibilities. For this purpose, three pure sulfated fucans from LH were tested; these fucans differed only in their molecular weight and were harvested at the same time, at the same place, with the same extraction method to achieve high comparability.

2. Results

2.1. Structural Characterization of the Sulfated Fucans

Monosaccharide anion-exchange chromatography of Fuc1 revealed a sugar composition of 97.0% ± 0.1% fucose (retention time 3.134 min) and 3.0% ± 0.1% galactose (retention time 7.910 min). Neither uronic acid residues nor glucose were detected.

Mass spectrometry of Fuc1 revealed a sulfite content ($-SO_3$) of 29.44%, which converts into a sulfation degree (DS) of approximately 1.7 sulfate groups per sugar residue (Table 1). Both (sugar composition and DS) are in full agreement with the previously elucidated molecular structure [12]. An overlay of the Raman spectra from samples Fuc1, Fuc2, and Fuc3 showed no change in the relative intensities of the sulfate group vibrations (822.5 cm^{-1}, 839.8 cm^{-1}, 1065.3 cm^{-1}, 1262.4 cm^{-1}) and methyl group vibrations (1340.9 cm^{-1}, 1452.5 cm^{-1}), indicating an equal ratio between the two groups and thereby showing that no desulfation occurred during the mild acid hydrolysis.

SEC-MALS (Size-exclusion chromatography-Multi-Angle Light Scattering) analysis of Fuc1 revealed a very high molecular weight average of M_w = 1548 (± 4.1) kDa [14], resulting in an average degree of polymerization (DP_n) of 3512, with an approximated average monosaccharide unit weight of 290 g/mol [12]. The molar mass was broadly distributed between 300 kDa and 7 MDa, displaying coherent results throughout different injected volumes (50 µL and 100 µL, c = 1 g/L, see Figure 1). The radius of gyration as the Z-average (R_z) was found to be 83.0 nm. The overall shape of the molecule was determined through an rms conformation plot (rms radius [nm] versus M [g/mol], see Figure 2), displaying a slope (b) of 0.66 and thus indicating an overall random coil shape of the molecule (sphere b = 0.3; random coil b = 0.5; rigid rod b = 1) [15]. Considering the previously reported high degree of branching of the molecule, while having obtained the same sugar composition and degree of sulfation as shown in Kopplin et al. (2018) [12], the obtained shape of a random coil for an LH sulfated fucan molecule 3 times bigger supports the previously suggested overall structure of a large, highly flexible main chain with short side chains. Fuc2 and Fuc3 showed almost identical structural features, only differing in their degree of polymerization.

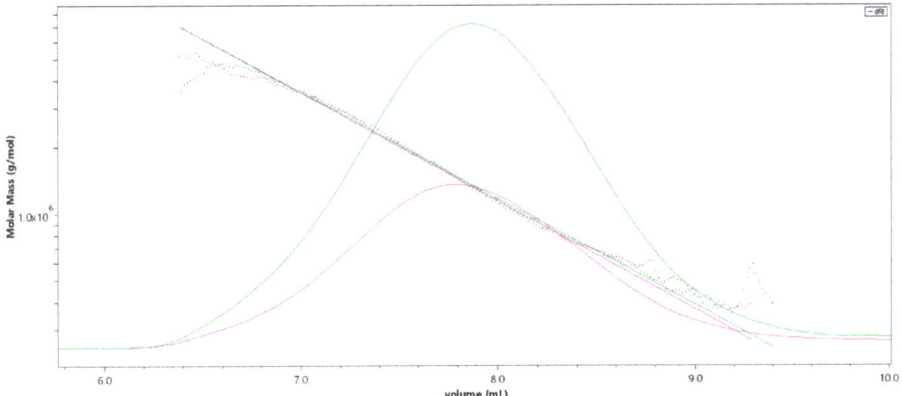

Figure 1. SEC-MALS (Size-exclusion chromatography-Multi-Angle Light Scattering) chromatogram of the high-molecular-weight sulfated fucan (Fuc1) giving M [g/mol] versus V [mL]; 50 µL injection (pink), 100 µL injection (green). The molar mass is plotted as a dotted line, the refractive index is displayed as an overlay.

Table 1. Data overview of the sulfated fucan samples used in this study. Degree of sulfation (DS), weight average molar mass (M_w), number average molar mass (M_n), degree of polymerization (DP), Z-average radius of gyration (R_z), refractive index increment (dn/dc), and slope of the RMS conformation plot (b = rms versus M).

	DS	M_w [kDa]	M_n [kDa]	DP_n	R_z [nm]	dn/dc	b
Fuc1	1.7	1548	1021	3512	83.0	0.115	0.66
Fuc2	1.7	499	241	829	47.1	0.115	0.66
Fuc3	1.7	26.9	13.9	48	-	0.115	-

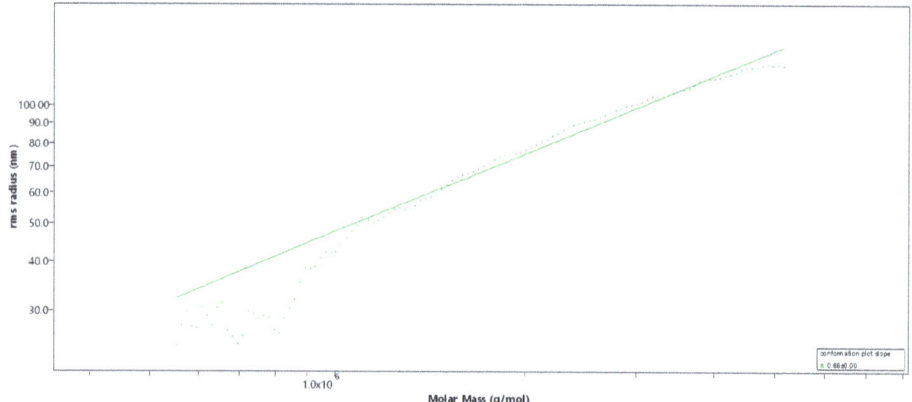

Figure 2. Rms conformation plot of the high-molecular-weight sulfated fucan (Fuc1) giving the rms radius [nm] versus M [g/mol], 100 μL injection. The slope (b) = 0.66 indicates a random coil.

2.2. Effects on Cell Viability

The uveal melanoma cell line OMM-1 was treated with the three LH sulfated fucans for 24 h; after that, an MTS (3-(4,5-Dimethylthiazol-2-yl)-5-(3-carboxymethoxyphenyl)-2-(4-sulfophenyl)-2H-tetrazolium) assay was conducted. In all three cases a dose-dependent decrease in cell viability starting with 1 μg/mL could be seen (Figure 3), but only Fuc2 and Fuc3 showed significant effects: 50 and 100 μg/mL Fuc2 lowered cell viability to 83% ± 5% ($p < 0.01$) and 76% ± 6% ($p < 0.001$), respectively. Quantities of 10, 50, and 100 μg/mL Fuc3 reduced cell viability even further to 87% ± 6%, 76% ± 5%, and 70% ± 9%, respectively. Fuc1, the sulfated fucan with the highest molecular weight, showed no significant effects on cell viability but showed a tendency at 100 μg/mL, which is not significant because of the higher variability.

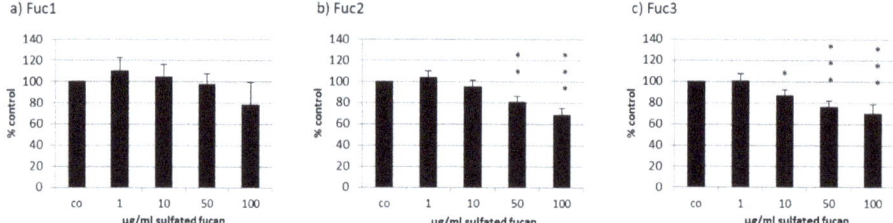

Figure 3. Cell viability was tested in uveal melanoma cell line OMM-1 after treatment with *Laminaria hyperborea* (LH) sulfated fucans Fuc1 (**a**), Fuc2 (**b**), and Fuc3 (**c**) for 24 h. Cell viability was determined via MTS (3-(4,5-Dimethylthiazol-2-yl)-5-(3-carboxymethoxyphenyl)-2-(4-sulfophenyl)-2H-tetrazolium) assay and is shown as the mean and standard deviation in relation to a 100% control. Significance was evaluated with ANOVA; * $p < 0.05$, ** $p < 0.01$, *** $p < 0.001$ compared to control ($n = 4$).

The human RPE cell line ARPE-19 was treated with the three LH sulfated fucans for 24 h and tested with a consecutive MTS assay. Only 50 μg/mL Fuc1 increased cell viability slightly (Figure 4).

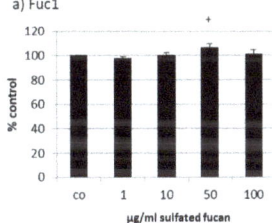
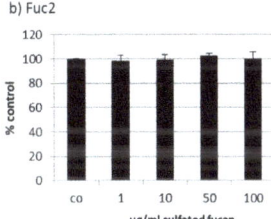
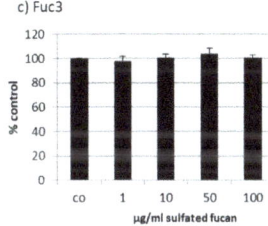

Figure 4. Cell viability was tested in retinal pigment epithelium (RPE) cell line ARPE-19 after treatment with LH sulfated fucans Fuc1 (**a**), Fuc2 (**b**), and Fuc3 (**c**) for 24 h. Cell viability was determined via MTS assay and is shown as the mean and standard deviation in relation to a 100% control. Significance was evaluated with ANOVA compared to the control ($n = 4$); $^{+}$ $p < 0.05$.

Primary porcine RPE cells were treated with the three LH sulfated fucans for 24 h and tested with an MTT (3-(4,5-dimethylthiazol-2-yl)-2,5-diphenyltetrazolium bromide) assay. The 10 µg/mL Fuc1 lowered viability slightly, but not to a biologically relevant degree (Figure 5). This paved the way for extended incubation times to measure VEGF secretion after 72 h (see below).

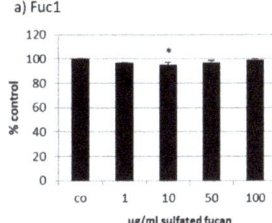
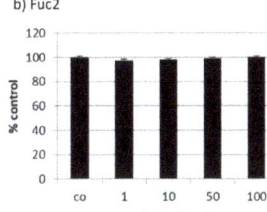
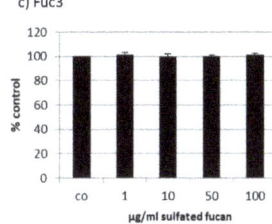

Figure 5. Cell viability was tested in RPE cells after treatment with LH sulfated fucans Fuc1 (**a**), Fuc2 (**b**), and Fuc3 (**c**) for 24 h. Cell viability was determined via MTT (3-(4,5-dimethylthiazol-2-yl)-2,5-diphenyltetrazolium bromide) assay and is shown as the mean and standard deviation in relation to an untreated control (100%). Significance was evaluated with ANOVA compared to the control ($n = 3$); * $p < 0.05$.

2.3. Oxidative Stress Protection

Oxidative stress protection by sulfated fucans from brown seaweed was already shown before for OMM-1 with *Fucus vesiculosus* sulfated fucan from Sigma-Aldrich [16] and with sulfated fucans from other seaweed, especially from SL, which was also protective for ARPE-19 [11]. So, these two cellular model systems are suitable for testing LH sulfated fucans.

Starting with the melanoma cell line OMM-1, stress induction with 1 mM H_2O_2 led to decreased cell viability of between 49% and 57% (Figure 6). The addition of 1–100 µg/mL Fuc2 showed no protection. The same outcome was achieved via treatment with Fuc3, which significantly reduced viability at 100 µg/mL (44% ± 9%, $p < 0.05$). Also, 50 µg/mL Fuc3 showed a slightly antiproliferative effect which was not significant. Only the sulfated fucan with the highest molecular weight, Fuc1, had significant protective effects at 10 µg/mL (65% ± 7%, $p < 0.05$).

RPE cells have the important role of protecting the cells of the retina against oxidative burden [7]. The RPE cell line ARPE19 was described to be rather resistant against hydrogen peroxide [17]. However, treatment with 0.5 mM *tert*-butyl hydroperoxide (TBHP) has a significant, consistent effect on the cell viability of ARPE-19 after 24 h, as previously shown [11].

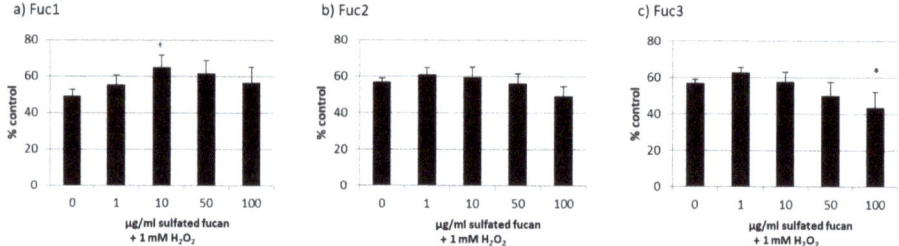

Figure 6. OMM-1 cell viability after treatment with Fuc1 (**a**), Fuc2 (**b**), and Fuc3 (**c**) and stress insult after 30 min incubation with the sulfated fucans. The oxidative agent was 1 mM H_2O_2, which reduced cell viability to under 60% in all cases. Viability was tested via MTS assay and is shown as the mean and standard deviation in relation to an untreated control (100%). The 10 µg/mL Fuc1 showed significant protective effects for the cell line. Significance was evaluated via ANOVA; */+ $p < 0.05$, versus 0 µg/mL sulfated fucan + 1 mM H_2O_2 ($n = 4$).

Cell viability was effectively lowered to nearly 30% through oxidative stress with TBHP, but all LH sulfated fucans lowered the viability additionally to a lesser extent (Figure 7); the strongest effect was from 100 µg/mL of the Fuc3 sulfated fucan, which lowered the viability even further down to 18% ± 1% ($p < 0.05$).

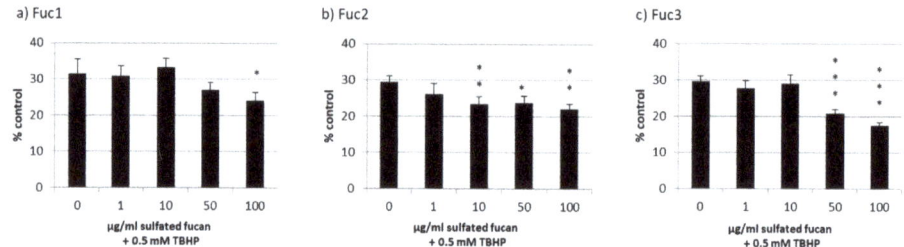

Figure 7. ARPE-19 cell viability after treatment with Fuc1 (**a**), Fuc2 (**b**), and Fuc3 (**c**) and stress insult after 30 min incubation with the sulfated fucans. The oxidative agent was 0.5 mM *tert*-butyl hydroperoxide (TBHP), which reduced cell viability to nearly 30% in all cases. Viability was tested via MTS assay and is shown as the mean and standard deviation in relation to an untreated control (100%). No sulfated fucan showed a significant protective effect for the RPE cell line. Significance was evaluated with ANOVA; * $p < 0.05$, ** $p < 0.01$, *** $p < 0.001$, versus 0 µg/mL sulfated fucan + 0.5 mM TBHP ($n = 4$).

2.4. VEGF Secretion

The effect of the three LH sulfated fucans on the secretion of VEGF was determined in the primary, porcine RPE cells and the human RPE cell line ARPE-19. ARPE-19 secreted nearly 4 times less VEGF compared to the primary RPE cells (ARPE-19: 66 pg/h and RPE: 243 pg/h). The VEGF content secreted into the supernatant of the cells was collected for ARPE-19 over 24 h and for RPE over 4 h because of the higher VEGF outcome. At this time point a medium exchange with added sulfated fucans was performed. The VEGF content [pg/mL] was normalized to the cell viability (after 72 h sulfated fucan treatment), giving the ratio of VEGF/cell viability (in arbitrary units [arb. unit]). The cell viability of both cell types with all sulfated fucans and all test concentrations was essentially unaffected (data not shown).

The secreted VEGF was lowered by all tested sulfated fucans in ARPE-19 (Figure 8). Fuc3 reduced VEGF to 0.84 ± 0.05 [arb. unit], $p < 0.001$, and Fuc2 lowered it to 0.66 ± 0.01 [arb. unit], $p < 0.001$, at 100 µg/mL. The effect of Fuc2 and Fuc3 on VEGF was concentration dependent. This did not apply for Fuc1, the sulfated fucan with the highest molecular weight, which reduced VEGF to 0.48 ± 0.04 [arb. unit], $p < 0.01$, at 50 µg/mL and had the strongest effect of all sulfated fucans at this concentration.

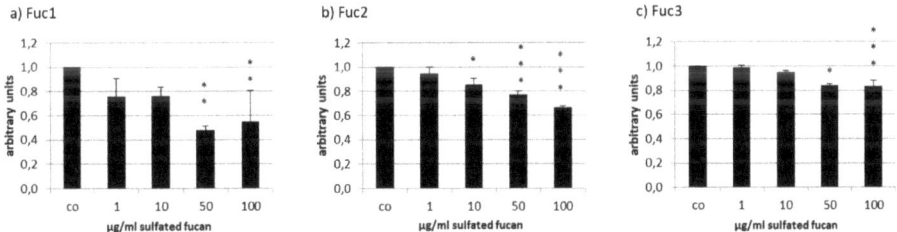

Figure 8. Vascular endothelial growth factor (VEGF) secretion of ARPE19 cells after incubation with Fuc1 (**a**), Fuc2 (**b**), and Fuc3 (**c**). VEGF content was analyzed with ELISA and normalized to cell viability. All LH extracts reduced VEGF content with 50 µg/mL Fuc1 as the most efficient. Significance was evaluated with ANOVA; * $p < 0.05$, ** $p < 0.01$, *** $p < 0.001$ compared to the control ($n = 4$).

Due to the high amount of VEGF production in RPE cells, weaker effects could be expected, but again VEGF was reduced by Fuc2 and Fuc1 (Figure 9). Fuc3, the smallest LH sulfated fucan, seemed to increased VEGF secretion at 10 µg/mL (1.21 ± 0.04 [arb. unit]); however, this change was not significant. Fuc2 reduced VEGF at 50 µg/mL to 0.64 ± 0.12 and at 100 µg/mL to 0.63 ± 0.10 [arb. unit], $p < 0.01$, and Fuc1 reduced VEGF at 50 µg/mL to 0.30 ± 0.09 [arb. unit], $p < 0.001$. Once more, Fuc1 had the highest efficiency and, similar to what was seen in ARPE-19, again showed the strongest effect at 50 µg/mL.

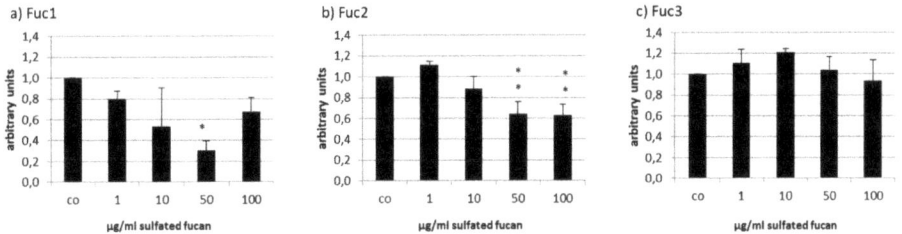

Figure 9. VEGF secretion of RPE cells after incubation with Fuc1 (**a**), Fuc2 (**b**), and Fuc3 (**c**). VEGF content was analyzed via ELISA and normalized to the cell viability. Fuc2 and Fuc1 reduced the VEGF content. Significance was evaluated via ANOVA; * $p < 0.05$, ** $p < 0.01$, compared to the control ($n = 3$).

3. Discussion

The different biological effects of sulfated fucans make them very interesting for medical research, but each sulfated fucan should be exactly characterized because of the high heterogeneity concerning these biological effects. Effects that are beneficial for the treatment of AMD were already described [2]. In this study we compared three purified sulfated fucans extracted from LH by Alginor ASA. The chemical structure was previously characterized and differs among the three samples only by the molecular weight average, which makes comparison in relation to the molecular weight possible. The aim was to prescreen these extracts as to whether they are suitable for further AMD-related research. To our knowledge, LH sulfated fucans had not been tested for this purpose before. Oxidative burden and VEGF secretion are two important factors in the risk of developing AMD and were therefore the main focus of this study. Because RPE cells are the target of the pathological mechanisms, they were chosen as the cellular models. The melanoma cell line OMM-1 acted as a model for oxidative stress protection as it is more susceptible to oxidative stress than the RPE cells.

First, the LH sulfated fucans were tested for their effects on the viability of primary RPE cells and the RPE cell line ARPE-19. In both cases there were no significant effects, which is in line with earlier studies like that by Bittkau et al. 2019, which reported that sulfated fucans in general are not antiproliferative for adherent cell lines [18]. However, this is dependent on the specific fucoidan and model system. For example Banafa et al. described antiproliferative effects of *Fucus vesiculosus* sulfated fucan in human breast cancer cells [19]. It was demonstrated that it arrests the cell cycle at G_1, has pro-apoptotic properties, and enhances ROS formation [19]. Fuc2 and Fuc3 showed cell viability lowering effects in the melanoma cell line OMM-1, which could be desirable for possible use in anticancer treatments. They both have a size below 500 kDa, so the effects could be connected to the molecular weight and structure. Possibly, these sulfated fucans interfere with fibronectin, disturbing the adherence of the tumor cell line [20]. Of note, the attachment of OMM-1 to well plates is rather weak and the cells have no tight junctions, in contrast to the RPE and ARPE-19 cell lines. In addition, OMM-1 cells were treated at subconfluence and the sulfated fucans could slow down the proliferation of this cell line, whereas the RPE cells were already confluent.

Because oxidative burden is considered one of the main causes of the development of AMD [7], the capability of the sulfated fucans to lower oxidative stress induced by TBHP or H_2O_2 was investigated. In ARPE-19, no protective effects could be detected, and 100 μg/mL Fuc3 had a cumulative toxic effect (also for OMM-1), which means that the smallest LH sulfated fucan enhanced the toxic effect of TBHP and H_2O_2. The same outcome was achieved for the OMM-1 cell line, except for the biggest sulfated fucan Fuc1, which was protective. These results are in contrast to those for the sulfated fucans of *Sargassum angustifolium*, in which the antioxidant activity through the scavenging of radicals and reducing power increased with decreasing size of the sulfated fucan (size range from 421 to 64 kDa) [21]. Because Fuc2 and Fuc3, which were also in that range, had no effect at all, and due to the absence of polyphenols by virtue of the high purity, it could be assumed that Fuc1 had no scavenging effect but rather interacted with the antioxidant defense system of the OMM-1 cell line. The RPE cells have an already improved antioxidant defense system, controlled via Nrf-2 (transcription factor nuclear factor erythroid 2-like 2), because of the high accumulation of oxygen radicals in the photoreceptors [7]. We already showed before that several sulfated fucans have protective effects in the OMM-1 cell line, but rarely do they in the ARPE-19 cell line [11,16]. OMM-1 cells have decreased superoxide dismutase activity [22], which could mean that the protective effects of ARPE-19 are concealed by already existing antioxidant enzyme activity. That sulfated fucans can activate superoxide dismutase and Nrf-2 was shown previously [23–26].

A further important factor, mainly for the development of wet AMD, is the secretion of VEGF, which supports the angiogenesis of blood vessels in the eye. ARPE-19 cell lines and the primary RPE cells were tested for their VEGF output after sulfated fucan treatment for three days. The secreted VEGF was normalized to the cell viability. As shown before, primary RPE cells produce significantly more VEGF compared to the cell line [11] (nearly 4 times more than ARPE-19); therefore, any significant reduction of the growth factor in primary RPE cells is even more remarkable. All three LH sulfated fucans decreased VEGF significantly at 50 and 100 μg/mL, with efficiency decreasing with smaller size in the RPE and ARPE-19 cells. This reducing effect could be due to the direct binding of VEGF, which inhibits the activation of the VEGF receptor. The negatively charged side chains of sulfated fucans can interact with the positively charged residues of the VEGF molecule, which could explain the interference in the binding between VEGF and its receptor [27]. This corresponds to findings in the literature [28,29]. It could be assumed that bigger size of the sulfated fucan is more efficient in VEGF inhibition. Also, direct interaction with the VEGF receptor (VEGF-R) [28] or the suppression of the VEGF and VEGF receptor genes could be possible, as VEGF has been shown to be involved in its own regulation [3,30–33]. Additional VEGF binding assays should be performed to determine the affinity of the fucoidan to the growth factor, which should be considered for further studies with LH sulfated fucans. Even more striking is the effect in the RPE cells, in which Fuc1 and Fuc2 also decreased VEGF despite the higher secretion. For both cell types, 50 μg/mL Fuc1 had the strongest effect. Fuc3 showed a tendency to stimulate VEGF secretion in RPE cells; however, this was not significant and its biological relevance is therefore uncertain. Nevertheless, it is of interest, as this small sulfated fucan may interact with VEGF differently to its high-molecular-weight counterpart, possibly by binding to VEGF in a VEGF-R-activating manner [34] The DS is also an important factor for the angiogenesis influencing effect [29], but the DS for all three sulfated fucans was the same.

The monosaccharide analysis by anion-exchange chromatography revealed a polysaccharide almost exclusively composed of fucose (97.0% fucose, 3.0% galactose). In addition, the sulfite content (-SO_3) of 29.44% (DS = 1.7) determined by ICP-MS is in strong agreement with data from the previously elucidated LH sulfated fucan structure [12]. The obtained rms conformation plot slope (b) of 0.66 through SEC-MALS revealed a random coil shape for both Fuc1 and Fuc2, further supporting the previously suggested long backbone structure (1→3 glycosidic linkages) with short side chains at 1→2 and 1→4 branching points. Therefore, the main difference between Fuc1, Fuc2, and Fuc3 was the degree of polymerization, directly associating the effects on proliferation, oxidative stress protection, and VEGF secretion with one structural property.

It has been shown that fucoidan, due to its high degree of sulfation, is able to bind to FGF (fibroblast growth factor) receptors, similar to heparin, heparan sulfate, and sulfated alginate [35–37]. Further has it been shown that the binding and inhibition of chemo- and cytokines, such as transforming growth factor-β1 (TGF-β1), by sulfated fucans is size dependent. Even though the underlying mechanism is not yet resolved, a similar binding preference could play a role [38].

Koyanagi et al. demonstrated that highly sulfated fucans are able to bind VEGF [29].

In addition, it has been found that polymers with conjugated inhibitors have a higher inhibitory effect on tumor necrosis factor-α (TNF-α) if the inhibitors are attached to higher-molecular-weight polymers; this is due to an increased diffusion time [39]. Since the binding of VEGF to highly sulfated fucans has been proven, a similar effect of increased diffusion time could play a role.

FCSP are a diverse group of macromolecules with heterogeneous molecular structures. Still, due to its almost exclusive fucose sugar composition and the full sulfation of almost every sugar unit, LH sulfated fucan is rather homogeneous in nature, even when hydrolyzed to different molecular weight averages. Hence, it can be speculated that biological effects on cells and the metabolism are less likely caused by chemical reaction or direct receptor interactions only expressed by Fuc1 and not Fuc2 and Fuc3, but rather by physical and steric interactions such as stronger cell surface adhesion or stronger entanglement with proteins (cadherins or cytokines) due to the higher average molecular weight.

For further clarification, other FCSP with similar M_w but lower DS [14] should be included in future studies, as well as high-molecular-weight hyaluronic acids, alginates, and sulfated alginates [40,41] to better elucidate and distinguish the effects caused by molecular size, charge density, and degree of sulfation and to determine if branching points and sugar composition play an additional role. Potential FCSP–cytokine binding needs to be investigated to exclude potential masking of the determined VEGF secretion. Finally, a chromatographic fractionation of high-molecular-weight LH sulfated fucan should be applied to narrow down the molecular weight range and the polydispersity and to get access to LH sulfated fucan fractions of even higher molecular weight, potentially amplifying the previously expressed effects and directly relating them to specific molecular weight ranges.

From the results taken together, the sulfated fucan Fuc1 from LH with a molecular weight average of 1548 kDa seems to be best candidate for further research concerning AMD-relevant mechanisms. It did not lower the cell viability of primary RPE cells, and 50 µg/mL inhibited VEGF most efficiently. High molecular weight appears to be desirable for VEGF inhibition. We tested several sulfated fucans from different algal species previously; sulfated fucans from SL were also effective in oxidative stress protection in the OMM-1 and ARPE-19 cell lines, and 10 µg/mL SL sulfated fucan inhibited VEGF in ARPE-19 and RPE cells [11]. The molecular weight for this sulfated fucan was 1407 kDa (unpublished data), so it is comparable to Fuc1, which also lowered VEGF significantly at 10 µg/mL in RPE and ARPE-19. This renders SL and LH sulfated fucans as promising candidates for further AMD-related studies. Of note, the pure LH sulfated fucan in this study can be sustainably reproduced in high amounts for further experiments in perfusion cultures or in vivo studies. Furthermore, because of its protective effect in the sensitive OMM-1 cell line, it could be considered for future studies with neuronal model systems concerning oxidative stress protection. For further research, tests concerning inflammation, lipid metabolism, and complement systems would be of additional interest.

4. Material and Methods

4.1. Cell Culture

The uveal melanoma cell line OMM-1 [42] was provided by Dr. Sarah Coupland. RPMI 1640 (Merck, Darmstadt, Germany) was used for cultivation (with 10% fetal calf serum (Linaris GmbH, Wertheim-Bettingen, Germany) and 1% penicillin/streptomycin (Merck, Darmstadt, Germany)).

The human RPE cell line ARPE-19 [43] was purchased from ATCC. The cultivation medium was HyClone DMEM (GE Healthcare, München, Germany) with 1% penicillin/streptomycin, 1.2% HEPES, 1% non-essential amino acids (all from Merck, Darmstadt, Germany), and 10% fetal calf serum, as previously described [11].

Primary porcine RPE cells were prepared as described before [30,44]. RPE cells were detached from porcine eyes by trypsin incubation and cultivated in HyClone DMEM (GE Healthcare, München, Germany) supplemented with penicillin/streptomycin (1%), HEPES (2.5%), non-essential amino acids (1%) (all Merck, Darmstadt, Germany), and 10% fetal calf serum.

ARPE-19 and RPE were treated at confluence, and OMM-1 cells were treated at subconfluence.

4.2. Sulfated Fucan

Extraction: Freshly frozen LH was thawed, blended into small particles (≤ 3 mm), and kept in 90 °C H_2O for 6 h. The solution was filtered (20–25 µm particle retention) using a vacuum pump; $CaCl_2$ was added to the filtrate and it was filtrated again (5 µm particle retention). The newly obtained filtrate was purified through ultrafiltration (300 kDa MWCO) and lyophilized.

Hydrolyzation: Lower-molecular-weight samples were obtained by mild acid hydrolysis of the ultrapurified sulfated fucan at pH = 3.0, 70 °C, and 5 min for Fuc2 and 35 min for Fuc3. The hydrolysates were cooled in ice water, dialyzed again with distilled water for 3 h (12 kDa MWCO), and lyophilized.

The purified and dried LH sulfated fucans Fuc1, Fuc2, and Fuc3 were dissolved in 5 mg/mL Ampuwa bidest (Fresenius, Schweinfurt, Germany). Before testing, the extracts were filtered with 0.2 µm Sarstedt filters (Nümbrecht, Germany) and further diluted in adequate medium to the concentrations mentioned in 4.6, 4.7, 4.8 and 4.9.

4.3. Monosaccharide Analysis

The sulfated fucan samples were hydrolyzed using 3 mol/L trifluoroacetic acid (TFA) at 95 °C for 12 h. The hydrolyzed monosaccharides were fractionated and analyzed through ion-exchange chromatography equipped with a CarboPac PA20 (Thermo Fisher Scientific Inc., Waltham, MA, USA) column.

4.4. Sulfate Content

The sulfate content of the ultrapurified sulfated fucan Fuc1 was externally analyzed using an Agilent 7500 Series quadrupole ICP-MS. The sulfate content of the hydrolyzed sulfated fucans was analyzed by Raman spectroscopy as previously described [12]. Raman spectra were recorded at room temperature using a Horiba Jobin–Yvon LabRAM HR system equipped with a Raman microscope (HORIBA Ltd., Kyoto, Japan).

4.5. Molecular Weight Determination

The molecular weight of the sulfated fucan was determined by size-exclusion chromatography (SEC) in the form of HPLC equipped with online multiangle static light scattering (MALS). The measurements were performed at ambient temperature using a Shodex LB-806 and a 2500 PWXL column as a separator. The measurement was executed with a Dawn HELEOS-8+ multiangle laser light scattering photometer (Wyatt, Santa Barbara, CA, USA) (λ_0 = 660 nm) and a subsequent Optilab T-rEX differential refractometer. The mobile phase was 0.10 mol/L Na_2HPO_4 (pH = 7), and the flow rate was 0.2 mL/min. The injection volumes were 50 µL and 100 µL, with 1 g/mL. The data were obtained and processed using Astra (v. 7) software (Wyatt, Santa Barbara, CA, USA).

4.6. Oxidative Stress

To induce oxidative-stress-related cell death, OMM-1 cells were treated with 1 mM H_2O_2 and ARPE-19 cells were treated with 500 µM TBHP as previously established [11,16] to reduce cell viability to nearly 50% (tested via MTS assay, see below). Before insult with the oxidative agents, cells were incubated with 1, 10, 50, and 100 µg/mL LH extracts.

4.7. Methyl Thiazolyl Tetrazolium (MTT) Assay

The widely used MTT assay [45] was conducted as previously described [4,11] and was used after taking supernatants for the VEGF ELISA (see below) and after 24 h sulfated fucan (1–100 µg/mL) stimulation. The cells were incubated with 0.5 mg/mL MTT for 2 h and dissolved in DMSO. Measurement was taken at 550 nm with an Elx800 (BioTek Instruments Inc., Bad Friedrichshall, Germany).

4.8. MTS Assay

The CellTiter 96® AQueous One Solution Cell Proliferation Assay from Promega Corporation (Mannheim, Germany) was used to measure the cell viability after 24 h treatment with 1–100 µg/mL LH extracts and in parallel to determine any protective effects after insult with oxidative stress. The abovementioned media and supplements were used without phenol red. To each well, 20 µl MTS was added, and the plates were incubated for 1 h.

4.9. VEGF ELISA

ARPE-19 and RPE supernatants were collected after treatment with LH extracts (1, 10, 50, and 100 µg/mL) on Day 3 after stimulation [11]. Medium with sulfated fucan was exchanged 24 h (ARPE-19) or 4 h (RPE) before collecting supernatants. Human VEGF DuoSet® ELISA was used for ARPE-19, whereas the Human VEGF Quantikine® ELISA was used for RPE supernatants (both R&D Systems, Wiesbaden, Germany). ELISAs were performed according to the manufacturer's instructions. Untreated cells and medium samples were tested as controls. To set the VEGF secretion in relation to the cell viability, MTT assay was conducted after collection of the supernatants on Day 3.

4.10. Statistics

Experiments were independently repeated at least three times. Statistics were calculated in Microsoft Excel (Excel 2010, Microsoft) and GraphPad PRISM 7 (GraphPad Software, Inc. 2017). p values of <0.05, calculated via ANOVA, were considered significant. The diagram bars and lines represent the mean and standard deviation, respectively.

5. Conclusions

The aim of this study was to investigate the effects of three pure sulfated fucans from *Laminaria hyperborea*, which differed in their molecular size. The sulfated fucan origin and extraction method were the same, and they differed only in the molecular weight average (Fuc1 > Fuc2 > Fuc3), paving the way for comparable data. To test whether they are suitable for further testing for potential treatment of, e.g., AMD, different tests regarding oxidative stress protection (MTS), cell viability (MTT/MTS), and VEGF interference (VEGF ELISA) in ocular cells (OMM-1, ARPE-19, and RPE) were performed. The cell viability of ARPE-19 and RPE was not influenced by up to three days of treatment; this is important for further studies because it excludes toxic effects. Fuc2 and Fuc3 lowered the cell viability of the melanoma cell line OMM-1 and should therefore be tested in further tumor cell lines as to whether this is cell line specific or in general for tumor cells, which could pave the way for anticancer studies. Fuc1, the biggest sulfated fucan, was the only one which showed protective effects against oxidative stress (in OMM-1). Fuc3 reduced VEGF secretion in ARPE19 but stimulated VEGF secretion in primary RPE cells. Conversely, Fuc2 and Fuc1 inhibited VEGF in ARPE-19 as well as in RPE, with the strongest effect seen for 50 µg/mL Fuc1. Altogether, the results showed that the biological activity of sulfated fucans is dependent on the molecular weight, and the desired effect for the treatment of ocular diseases increases with the size of the sulfated fucan.

Author Contributions: Conceptualization, A.K., G.K.; Methodology, A.K., G.K., P.D.; Validation, P.D.; Formal Analysis, P.D.; Investigation, G.K., P.D.; Resources, A.K., G.K., J.R.; Data Curation, A.K., P.D.; Writing—Original Draft Preparation, G.K., P.D.; Writing—Review and Editing, A.K., G.K., P.D.; Visualization, G.K., P.D.; Supervision, A.K., J.R.

Funding: This study is part of the FucoSan—Health from the Sea Project and is supported by EU InterReg–Deutschland–Denmark and the European Fund of Regional Development.

Acknowledgments: We thank Alginor ASA for the provision of the algae.

Conflicts of Interest: The authors declare no conflict of interest.

References

1. Deniaud-Bouët, E.; Hardouin, K.; Potin, P.; Kloareg, B.; Hervé, C. A review about brown algal cell walls and fucose-containing sulfated polysaccharides: Cell wall context, biomedical properties and key research challenges. *Carbohydr. Polym.* **2017**, *175*, 395–408. [CrossRef]
2. Li, B.; Lu, F.; Wei, X.; Zhao, R. Fucoidan: Structure and bioactivity. *Molecules* **2008**, *13*, 1671–1695. [CrossRef] [PubMed]
3. Klettner, A. Fucoidan as a Potential Therapeutic for Major Blinding Diseases—A Hypothesis. *Mar. Drugs* **2016**, *14*, 31. [CrossRef] [PubMed]
4. Dithmer, M.; Fuchs, S.; Shi, Y.; Schmidt, H.; Richert, E.; Roider, J.; Klettner, A. Fucoidan reduces secretion and expression of vascular endothelial growth factor in the retinal pigment epithelium and reduces angiogenesis in vitro. *PLoS ONE* **2014**, *9*, e89150. [CrossRef] [PubMed]
5. Miller, J.W. Age-related macular degeneration revisited—piecing the puzzle: The LXIX Edward Jackson memorial lecture. *Am. J. Ophthalmol.* **2013**, *155*, 1–35.e13. [CrossRef] [PubMed]
6. Ding, X.; Patel, M.; Chan, C.-C. Molecular pathology of age-related macular degeneration. *Prog. Retin. Eye Res.* **2009**, *28*, 1–18. [CrossRef] [PubMed]
7. Klettner, A. Oxidative stress induced cellular signaling in RPE cells. *Front. Biosci.* **2012**, *4*, 392–411. [CrossRef]
8. Hageman, G.S.; Anderson, D.H.; Johnson, L.V.; Hancox, L.S.; Taiber, A.J.; Hardisty, L.I.; Hageman, J.L.; Stockman, H.A.; Borchardt, J.D.; Gehrs, K.M.; et al. A common haplotype in the complement regulatory gene factor H (HF1/CFH) predisposes individuals to age-related macular degeneration. *Proc. Natl. Acad. Sci. USA* **2005**, *102*, 7227–7232. [CrossRef] [PubMed]
9. McHarg, S.; Clark, S.J.; Day, A.J.; Bishop, P.N. Age-related macular degeneration and the role of the complement system. *Mol. Immunol.* **2015**, *67*, 43–50. [CrossRef] [PubMed]
10. Schmidt-Erfurth, U.; Chong, V.; Loewenstein, A.; Larsen, M.; Souied, E.; Schlingemann, R.; Eldem, B.; Monés, J.; Richard, G.; Bandello, F. Guidelines for the management of neovascular age-related macular degeneration by the European Society of Retina Specialists (EURETINA). *Br. J. Ophthalmol.* **2014**, *98*, 1144–1167. [CrossRef] [PubMed]
11. Dörschmann, P.; Bittkau, K.S.; Neupane, S.; Roider, J.; Alban, S.; Klettner, A. Effects of fucoidans from five different brown algae on oxidative stress and VEGF interference in ocular cells. *Mar. Drugs* **2019**, *17*, 258. [CrossRef] [PubMed]

12. Kopplin, G.; Rokstad, A.M.; Mélida, H.; Bulone, V.; Skjåk-Bræk, G.; Aachmann, F.L. Structural Characterization of Fucoidan from Laminaria hyperborea: Assessment of Coagulation and Inflammatory Properties and Their Structure–Function Relationship. *ACS Appl. Bio Mater.* **2018**, *1*, 1880–1892. [CrossRef]
13. Stefaniak–Vidarsson, M.M.; Gudjónsdóttir, M.; Marteinsdottir, G.; Sigurjonsson, O.E.; Kristbergsson, K. Evaluation of bioactivity of fucoidan from laminaria with in vitro human cell cultures (THP-1). *Funct. Foods Health Dis.* **2017**, *7*, 688. [CrossRef]
14. Fitton, J.H.; Stringer, D.N.; Karpiniec, S.S. Therapies from Fucoidan: An Update. *Mar. Drugs* **2015**, *13*, 5920–5946. [CrossRef] [PubMed]
15. Smidsrød, O.; Moe, S. *Biopolymer Chemistry*, 2nd ed.; Tapir Academic Press: Trondheim, Norway, 2008.
16. Dithmer, M.; Kirsch, A.-M.; Richert, E.; Fuchs, S.; Wang, F.; Schmidt, H.; Coupland, S.E.; Roider, J.; Klettner, A. Fucoidan Does Not Exert Anti-Tumorigenic Effects on Uveal Melanoma Cell Lines. *Mar. Drugs* **2017**, *15*, 193. [CrossRef] [PubMed]
17. Karlsson, M.; Kurz, T. Attenuation of iron-binding proteins in ARPE-19 cells reduces their resistance to oxidative stress. *Acta Ophthalmol.* **2016**, *94*, 556–564. [CrossRef] [PubMed]
18. Bittkau, K.S.; Dörschmann, P.; Blümel, M.; Tasdemir, D.; Roider, J.; Klettner, A.; Alban, S. Comparison of the Effects of Fucoidans on the Cell Viability of Tumor and Non-Tumor Cell Lines. *Mar. Drugs* **2019**, *17*, 441. [CrossRef]
19. Banafa, A.M.; Roshan, S.; Liu, Y.-Y.; Chen, H.-J.; Chen, M.-J.; Yang, G.-X.; He, G.-Y. Fucoidan induces G1 phase arrest and apoptosis through caspases-dependent pathway and ROS induction in human breast cancer MCF-7 cells. *J. Huazhong Univ. Sci. Technol.* **2013**, *33*, 717–724. [CrossRef]
20. Liu, J.M.; Bignon, J.; Haroun-Bouhedia, F.; Bittoun, P.; Vassy, J.; Fermandjian, S.; Wdzieczak-Bakala, J.; Boisson-Vidal, C. Inhibitory Effect of Fucoidan on the Adhesion of Adenocarcinoma Cells to Fibronectin. *Anticancer Res.* **2005**, *25*, 2129–2134.
21. Borazjani, N.J.; Tabarsa, M.; You, S.; Rezaei, M. Improved immunomodulatory and antioxidant properties of unrefined fucoidans from Sargassum angustifolium by hydrolysis. *J. Food Sci. Technol.* **2017**, *54*, 4016–4025. [CrossRef]
22. Blasi, M.A.; Maresca, V.; Roccella, M.; Roccella, F.; Sansolini, T.; Grammatico, P.; Balestrazzi, E.; Picardo, M. Antioxidant pattern in uveal melanocytes and melanoma cell cultures. *Investig. Ophthalmol. Vis. Sci.* **1999**, *40*, 3012–3016.
23. Foresti, R.; Bucolo, C.; Platania, C.M.B.; Drago, F.; Dubois-Randé, J.-L.; Motterlini, R. Nrf2 activators modulate oxidative stress responses and bioenergetic profiles of human retinal epithelial cells cultured in normal or high glucose conditions. *Pharmacol. Res.* **2015**, *99*, 296–307. [CrossRef] [PubMed]
24. Ryu, M.J.; Chung, H.S. Fucoidan reduces oxidative stress by regulating the gene expression of HO-1 and SOD-1 through the Nrf2/ERK signaling pathway in HaCaT cells. *Mol. Med. Rep.* **2016**, *14*, 3255–3260. [CrossRef] [PubMed]
25. Vomund, S.; Schäfer, A.; Parnham, M.J.; Brüne, B.; von Knethen, A. Nrf2, the Master Regulator of Anti-Oxidative Responses. *Int. J. Mol. Sci.* **2017**, *18*, 2772. [CrossRef] [PubMed]
26. Wang, Y.-Q.; Wei, J.-G.; Tu, M.-J.; Gu, J.-G.; Zhang, W. Fucoidan Alleviates Acetaminophen-Induced Hepatotoxicity via Oxidative Stress Inhibition and Nrf2 Translocation. *Int. J. Mol. Sci.* **2018**, *19*, 4050. [CrossRef] [PubMed]
27. Marinval, N.; Saboural, P.; Haddad, O.; Maire, M.; Bassand, K.; Geinguenaud, F.; Djaker, N.; Ben Akrout, K.; La Lamy de Chapelle, M.; Robert, R.; et al. Identification of a Pro-Angiogenic Potential and Cellular Uptake Mechanism of a LMW Highly Sulfated Fraction of Fucoidan from Ascophyllum nodosum. *Mar. Drugs* **2016**, *14*, 185. [CrossRef] [PubMed]
28. Chen, H.; Cong, Q.; Du, Z.; Liao, W.; Zhang, L.; Yao, Y.; Ding, K. Sulfated fucoidan FP08S2 inhibits lung cancer cell growth in vivo by disrupting angiogenesis via targeting VEGFR2/VEGF and blocking VEGFR2/Erk/VEGF signaling. *Cancer Lett.* **2016**, *382*, 44–52. [CrossRef] [PubMed]
29. Koyanagi, S.; Tanigawa, N.; Nakagawa, H.; Soeda, S.; Shimeno, H. Oversulfation of fucoidan enhances its anti-angiogenic and antitumor activities. *Biochem. Pharmacol.* **2003**, *65*, 173–179. [CrossRef]
30. Klettner, A.; Roider, J. Comparison of bevacizumab, ranibizumab, and pegaptanib in vitro: Efficiency and possible additional pathways. *Investig. Ophthalmol. Vis. Sci.* **2008**, *49*, 4523–4527. [CrossRef]

31. Klettner, A.; Westhues, D.; Lassen, J.; Bartsch, S.; Roider, J. Regulation of constitutive vascular endothelial growth factor secretion in retinal pigment epithelium/choroid organ cultures, P38, nuclear factor κB, and the vascular endothelial growth factor receptor-2/phosphatidylinositol 3 kinase pathway. *Mol. Vis.* **2013**, *19*, 281–291.
32. Liu, F.; Wang, J.; Chang, A.K.; Liu, B.; Yang, L.; Li, Q.; Wang, P.; Zou, X. Fucoidan extract derived from Undaria pinnatifida inhibits angiogenesis by human umbilical vein endothelial cells. *Phytomedicine* **2012**, *19*, 797–803. [CrossRef] [PubMed]
33. Narazaki, M.; Segarra, M.; Tosato, G. Sulfated polysaccharides identified as inducers of neuropilin-1 internalization and functional inhibition of VEGF165 and semaphorin3A. *Blood* **2008**, *111*, 4126–4136. [CrossRef] [PubMed]
34. Lake, A.C.; Vassy, R.; Di Benedetto, M.; Lavigne, D.; Le Visage, C.; Perret, G.Y.; Letourneur, D. Low molecular weight fucoidan increases VEGF165-induced endothelial cell migration by enhancing VEGF165 binding to VEGFR-2 and NRP1. *J. Biol. Chem.* **2006**, *281*, 37844–37852. [CrossRef] [PubMed]
35. Foxall, C.; Wei, Z.; Schaefer, M.E.; Casabonne, M.; Fugedi, P.; Peto, C.; Castellot, J.J.; Brandley, B.K. Sulfated malto-oligosaccharides bind to basic FGF, inhibit endothelial cell proliferation, and disrupt endothelial cell tube formation. *J. Cell. Physiol.* **1996**, *168*, 657–667. [CrossRef]
36. Kwak, J.-Y. Fucoidan as a marine anticancer agent in preclinical development. *Mar. Drugs* **2014**, *12*, 851–870. [CrossRef] [PubMed]
37. Arlov, Ø.; Aachmann, F.L.; Feyzi, E.; Sundan, A.; Skjåk-Bræk, G. The Impact of Chain Length and Flexibility in the Interaction between Sulfated Alginates and HGF and FGF-2. *Biomacromolecules* **2015**, *16*, 3417–3424. [CrossRef] [PubMed]
38. Kim, T.H.; Lee, E.K.; Lee, M.J.; Kim, J.H.; Yang, W.S. Fucoidan inhibits activation and receptor binding of transforming growth factor-β1. *Biochem. Biophys. Res. Commun.* **2013**, *432*, 163–168. [CrossRef] [PubMed]
39. Washburn, N.R.; Prata, J.E.; Friedrich, E.E.; Ramadan, M.H.; Elder, A.N.; Sun, L.T. Polymer-conjugated inhibitors of tumor necrosis factor-α for local control of inflammation. *Biomatter* **2013**, *3*, e25597. [CrossRef] [PubMed]
40. Rayahin, J.E.; Buhrman, J.S.; Zhang, Y.; Koh, T.J.; Gemeinhart, R.A. High and low molecular weight hyaluronic acid differentially influence macrophage activation. *ACS Biomater. Sci. Eng.* **2015**, *1*, 481–493. [CrossRef]
41. Arlov, Ø.; Skjåk-Bræk, G.; Rokstad, A.M. Sulfated alginate microspheres associate with factor H and dampen the inflammatory cytokine response. *Acta Biomater.* **2016**, *42*, 180–188. [CrossRef]
42. Luyten, G.P.; Naus, N.C.; Mooy, C.M.; Hagemeijer, A.; Kan-Mitchell, J.; van Drunen, E.; Vuzevski, V.; de Jong, P.T.; Luider, T.M. Establishment and characterization of primary and metastatic uveal melanoma cell lines. *Int. J. Cancer* **1996**, *66*, 380–387. [CrossRef]
43. Dunn, K.C.; Aotaki-Keen, A.E.; Putkey, F.R.; Hjelmeland, L.M. ARPE-19, a human retinal pigment epithelial cell line with differentiated properties. *Exp. Eye Res.* **1996**, *62*, 155–169. [CrossRef] [PubMed]
44. Wiencke, A.K.; Kiilgaard, J.F.; Nicolini, J.; Bundgaard, M.; Röpke, C.; La Cour, M. Growth of cultured porcine retinal pigment epithelial cells. *Acta Ophthalmol. Scand.* **2003**, *81*, 170–176. [CrossRef] [PubMed]
45. Riss, T.L.; Moravec, R.A.; Niles, A.L.; Duellman, S.; Benink, H.A.; Worzella, T.J.; Minor, L. Cell Viability Assays. In *Assay Guidance Manual [Internet]*; Sittampalam, G.S., Coussens, N.P., Brimacombe, K., Grossman, A., Arkin, M., Auld, D., Austin, C., Baell, J., Bejcek, B., Caaveiro, J.M.M., et al., Eds.; Eli Lilly & Company and the National Center for Advancing Translational Sciences: Indianapolis, IN, USA, 2016.

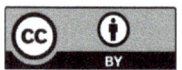

© 2019 by the authors. Licensee MDPI, Basel, Switzerland. This article is an open access article distributed under the terms and conditions of the Creative Commons Attribution (CC BY) license (http://creativecommons.org/licenses/by/4.0/).

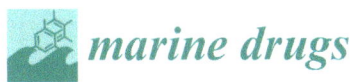

Article

The Inhibitory Effect of Propylene Glycol Alginate Sodium Sulfate on Fibroblast Growth Factor 2-Mediated Angiogenesis and Invasion in Murine Melanoma B16-F10 Cells In Vitro

He Ma [1], Peiju Qiu [1,2,3,4,*], Huixin Xu [1], Ximing Xu [1,2,3,4], Meng Xin [1,2,3,4], Yanyan Chu [1,2,3,4], Huashi Guan [1,2,3,4], Chunxia Li [1,3] and Jinbo Yang [1,2,3,4,*]

[1] Key Laboratory of Marine Drugs of Ministry of Education, Shandong Provincial, Key Laboratory of Glycoscience and Glycotechnology, School of Medicine and Pharmacy, Ocean University of China, Qingdao 266003, China; mahe1992mahe@163.com (H.M.); xvhuixin@hotmail.com (H.X.); xuximing@ouc.edu.cn (X.X.); xinmeng512@126.com (M.X.); mary0312332@126.com (Y.C.); hsguan@ouc.edu.cn (H.G.); lchunxia@ouc.edu.cn (C.L.)

[2] Innovation Center for Marine Drug Screening & Evaluation, Pilot National Laboratory for Marine Science and Technology (Qingdao), Qingdao 266237, China

[3] Laboratory for Marine Drugs and Bioproducts of Pilot National Laboratory for Marine Science and Technology (Qingdao), Qingdao 266237, China

[4] Marine Biomedical Research Institute of Qingdao, Qingdao 266071, China

* Correspondence: peijuqiu@ouc.edu.cn (P.Q.); yangjb@ouc.edu.cn (J.Y.); Tel.: +86-532-85906859 (P.Q.); +86-532-82032030 (J.Y.)

Received: 5 March 2019; Accepted: 23 April 2019; Published: 29 April 2019

Abstract: Melanoma is one of the most malignant and aggressive types of cancer worldwide. Fibroblast growth factor 2 (FGF2) is one of the critical regulators of melanoma angiogenesis and metastasis; thus, it might be an effective anti-cancer strategy to explore FGF2-targeting drug candidates from existing drugs. In this study, we evaluate the effect of the marine drug propylene glycol alginate sodium sulfate (PSS) on FGF2-mediated angiogenesis and invasion. The data shows that FGF2 selectively bound to PSS with high affinity. PSS inhibited FGF2-mediated angiogenesis in a rat aortic ring model and suppressed FGF2-mediated invasion, but not the migration of murine melanoma B16-F10 cells. The further mechanism study indicates that PSS decreased the expression of activated matrix metalloproteinase 2 (MMP-2) and matrix metalloproteinase 9 (MMP-9), and also suppressed their activity. In addition, PSS was found to decrease the level of Vimentin in B16-F10 cells, which is known to participate in the epithelial–mesenchymal transition. Notably, PSS did not elicit any changes in cancer cell viability. Based on the results above, we conclude that PSS might be a potential drug to regulate the tumor microenvironment in order to facilitate the recovery of melanoma patients.

Keywords: propylene glycol alginate sodium sulfate; angiogenesis; invasion; FGF2; MMP-2; MMP-9

1. Introduction

Melanoma is one of the most malignant and aggressive types of cancer worldwide, and the identification of new targets for treating melanoma is urgently needed. Melanoma cells have been reported to constitutively express fibroblast growth factor 2 (FGF2) [1,2], which is an autocrine factor and promotes the proliferation, angiogenesis, and metastasis of melanoma cells. Thus, FGF2 is commonly considered one of the potential targets for treating melanoma, and may be used with other targets to synergistically enhance therapeutic efficacy [3].

FGF2, which belongs to the FGF family, participates in a variety of physiological and pathological processes both in vitro and in vivo, including cellular survival, differentiation, proliferation, angiogenesis, adhesion, skeletal formation, and wound healing [4–6]. In terms of function, FGF2 first binds to two fibroblast growth factor receptors (FGFRs), and then recruits the heparan sulfate (HS) chain(s) of membrane-anchored heparan sulfate proteoglycan (HSPGs) for assembly into a ternary complex (FGF–HS–FGFR). The FGF–HS–FGFR complex results in receptor dimerization, with subsequent autophosphorylation of specific tyrosine residues that affects multiple downstream signal transduction pathways [7–10]. Meanwhile, FGF2 and FGFR-1 complexes can enter into the nucleus, where they engage with a variety of sequence-specific transcription factors and further regulate the release and activity of matrix metalloproteinase 2 (MMP-2) and matrix metalloproteinase 9 (MMP-9), as well as the expression of proteins involved in the epithelial–mesenchymal transition [11,12].

Among the FGF–HS–FGFR complex, the basic amino acid residues of FGF2–FGFR2 form a positively charged cluster, which can attract negatively-charged HS chains for incorporation. Exogenous sulfated carbohydrates like heparin and its mimetic derivatives have long been studied for their competition with HS chains, to break the formation of the FGF2–HS–FGFR1 ternary complex and physiologically disrupt the function of cancer cells [13]. Several heparin mimics have been proven to be effective in blocking the formation of the FGF2–HS–FGFR1 ternary complex in vitro; however, their potential use might be limited by their potency, pharmacokinetic defect, and safety profile. Therefore, it would be an effective strategy to explore FGF2 inhibitors from existing drugs to facilitate cancer treatment.

Propylene glycol alginate sodium sulfate (PSS) is a heparin-like drug that was approved by the China Food and Drug Administration (CFDA) over 30 years ago to treat hyperlipidemia and ischemic cardio-cerebrovascular diseases [14]. PSS is obtained from alginate polysaccharide of Laminaria with multiple chemical modifications. PSS is composed of mannuronic acid (M) and guluronic acid (G) disaccharide repeat units and sulfates occurring at the C-2 or C-3 position of the sugar moiety, with a substitution at the C-6 position by propylene glycol. PSS has the following structural characteristics: an M/G ratio above 1.5, a molecular weight of 15–20 kDa, and an organic sulfur content of 9–14% [15].

Based on our previous research, it is well known that PSS and its fractions exert effects on anti-coagulation-related activities and anti-selectin activities [15–17]. Wu et al. reported that PSS and its oligosaccharides could significantly stimulate FGF2-induced cell proliferation in FGFR1c-expressing BaF3 murine pro-B cell line [18], suggesting that the potential binding effect occurs between PSS and FGF2. However, no studies have investigated the effects of PSS on FGF2-mediated functional regulation on a highly metastatic B16-F10 melanoma model and the related tumor microenvironment. As PSS possesses similar structural and bioactive properties to heparin, we hypothesized that PSS might exhibit an inhibitory effect on FGF2-mediated cellular proliferation, invasion, migration, or angiogenesis, as well as related downstream signaling.

2. Results

2.1. Fibroblast Growth Factor 2 Bound to Propylene Glycol Alginate Sodium Sulfate with High Affinity

PSS was investigated by surface plasmon resonance (SPR) analysis for its affinity with FGF2 and vascular endothelial growth factor 165 (VEGF165). As shown in Figure 1, PSS bound directly to FGF2, and the equilibrium dissociation constant (KD) was 2.73×10^{-8} M, which is comparable to heparin (2.76×10^{-8} M). In contrast, weak affinity was detected between PSS and VEGF165 (Supplementary Table S1), while the KD of heparin was 8.09×10^{-7} M. As FGF2 is a crucial growth factor to regulate angiogenesis and the function of tumor cells, these data indicate that FGF2 was probably a potential target for PSS to improve tumor environment.

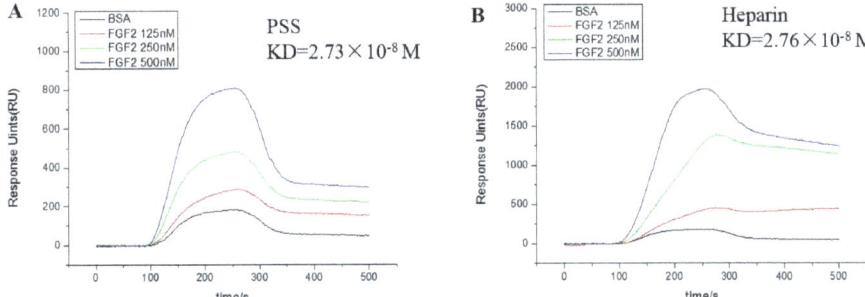

Figure 1. Analysis of the affinity between propylene glycol alginate sodium sulfate (PSS) and fibroblast growth factor 2 (FGF2). (**A**,**B**) were binding response curves of PSS and heparin with FGF2, respectively. PSS or Heparin (1–5 mM) was immobilized on Graft-to-PCL sensor chips. The mobile phase was FGF2 solution (dissolved in phosphate buffer solution (PBS)), and the concentrations were 125, 250, and 500 nM. The data obtained were analyzed and fitted by a PLEXERA SPR Data Analysis Module (DAM) to obtain the equilibrium dissociation constant (K_D). Images are representative of three independent experiments with similar results.

2.2. Propylene Glycol Alginate Sodium Sulfate Inhibited the Fibroblast Growth Factor 2-Induced Invasion of B16-F10 Cells

FGF2 has been reported to play an important role in tumor metastasis; thus, we next wanted to evaluate the role of PSS in inhibiting tumor cell invasion and metastasis. PSS significantly inhibited the serum-induced invasion of B16-F10 in a dose-dependent manner. The Matrigel barrier approach was used to evaluate tumor cell metastasis. As shown in Figure 2A,B, after treating the cells for 16 h, PSS inhibited invasion by 33.8%, 45.7%, and 61.8% at concentrations of 25, 50, and 100 µg/mL, respectively, in a dose-dependent manner. We further detected the anti-invasive effect of PSS on FGF2-mediated invasion. As shown in Figure 2C,D, 10% FBS and 200 ng/mL FGF2 induced a comparable number of B16-F10 cells to penetrate the growth factor-reduced Matrigel, and PSS significantly inhibited FGF2-induced invasion by 59.1% at a concentration of 50 µg/mL after treating the cells for 8 h.

2.3. Propylene Glycol Alginate Sodium Sulfate Had No Effect on Cell Viability

To ensure that the inhibitory effect of PSS on invasion was not due to the direct killing of tumor cells by PSS, we detected the proliferation ability of tumor cells after treatment with PSS for 48 h. No inhibition on proliferation was observed, even when the concentration was more than 1000 µg/mL (Figure 3), suggesting that the inhibitory effect of PSS on invasion was not due to a reduction in the viability of cancer cells, but was likely due to the inhibition of tumor cell migration or the suppression of matrix-degrading enzymes.

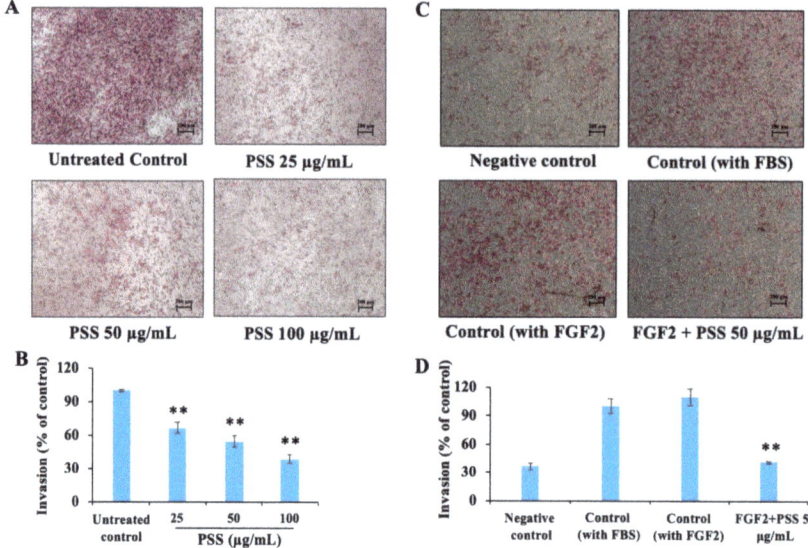

Figure 2. The effect of PSS on the invasion of B16-F10 cells. B16-F10 cells (1.5×10^4 cells/well) were seeded onto a membrane coated with Matrigel (**A,B**) or growth factor-reduced Matrigel (**C,D**), and were treated with various concentrations of PSS (25, 50, 100 µg/mL) for 16 h or 8 h (FGF2-mediated invasion of B16-F10). Cells that penetrated through to the lower surface of the membrane were stained with crystal violet and photographed under a light microscope at 40× magnification. Then, crystal violet was dissolved in 10% acetic acid, and the absorbance of the resulting solution was measured at 600 nm using a microplate reader (SpetraMAX i3, Molecular Devices, Sunnyvale, CA, USA). The controls included a negative control, complete medium only; control (with 10% FBS) complete medium with 10% FBS; control (with FGF2) complete medium with 200 ng/mL FGF2; and FGF2 + PSS 50 µg/mL complete medium with 200 ng/mL FGF2 and 50 µg/mL PSS. The results are from three independent experiments. ** $p < 0.01$, significant difference between PSS-treated groups and the untreated control by Student's t-test.

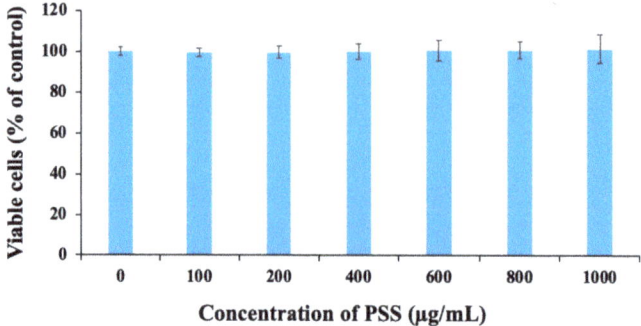

Figure 3. The effect of PSS on cell viability. B16-F10 cells (0.5×10^4 cells/well) were seeded in 96-well plates and incubated for 24 h to allow adherence. Various concentrations of PSS were added to the plates, and then the cells were further incubated for another 48 h. The resazurin assay (1 mg/mL) was used for detection. The absorbance of each well was measured at 405 nm by a microplate reader (SpetraMAX i3, Molecular Devices, Sunnyvale, CA, USA). The data obtained are from three independent experiments.

2.4. Propylene Glycol Alginate Sodium Sulfate Had No Effect on the Migration of B16-F10 Cells

Based on the results above, we further detected the effect of PSS on the migration of B16-F10 cells. As shown in Figure 4A,B, no obvious difference in the number of the migratory cells was found between the untreated control and the treatment with PSS at 400 µg/mL. Meanwhile, the results of the scratch wound migration assays also revealed no significant difference across the wounded region after treatment with PSS at 400 µg/mL for 24 h (Figure 4C). PSS also had no effect on the migration of human umbilical vein endothelial (HUVEC) cells (Supplementary Figure S1).

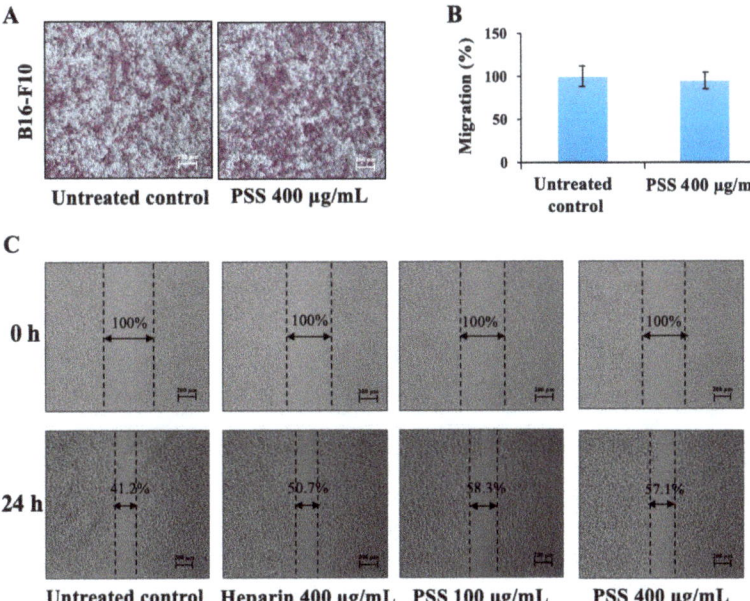

Figure 4. The effect of PSS on the migration of B16-F10 cells. B16-F10 cells (1×10^4 cells/well) were seeded into the upper chamber of Transwell plates, treated with various concentrations of PSS, and allowed to migrate for 16 h. Cells that penetrated through to the lower surface of the membrane were stained with crystal violet and photographed under a light microscope at 40× magnification (**A**). Then, crystal violet was dissolved in 10% acetic acid, and the absorbance of the resulting solution was measured at 600 nm using a microplate reader (SpetraMAX i3, Molecular Devices, Sunnyvale, CA, USA) (**B**). For the wound healing assay (**C**), 70% confluency B16-F10 cells in 12-well culture plates were scratched and then treated with FBS-free medium with PSS (100, 400 µg/mL) or 400 µg/mL heparin. Three randomly selected views along the wound line in each well were photographed under an inverted microscope at 0 h and 24 h after incubation. The percentage of void area with respect to time 0 was determined using ImageJ software (ImageJ 1.8.0, Rawak Software Inc., Stuttgart, Germany). The results are from three independent experiments. ** $p < 0.01$, significant difference between the PSS-treated groups and the untreated control by Student's t-test.

2.5. Propylene Glycol Alginate Sodium Sulfate Down-Regulated the Expression of Activated Matrix Metalloproteinase 2 and Matrix Metalloproteinase 9

The process of invasion involves the degradation of the ECM and the subsequent migration of tumor cells. Based on the data above, we confirmed that PSS inhibited the invasion of B16-F10 cells in a dose-dependent manner, but had no effect on tumor cell migration. Therefore, we examined whether PSS affected the expression or activity of crucial ECM-degrading enzymes. MMP-2 and MMP-9 are capable of degrading type IV collagen, which is the most abundant component of the basement membrane. Degradation of the basement membrane is an essential step for the metastatic progression of most cancers. Matrigel is an analog of the basement membrane. PSS inhibits the degradation of Matrigel by B16-F10. Therefore, it is necessary to detect whether PSS inhibits the expression and activity of MMP-2 and MMP-9. We first detected the effect of PSS on the expression of MMP-2 and MMP-9. After treating B16-F10 cells for 24 h, PSS was found to decrease the expression of activated MMP-2 in a dose-dependent manner. PSS inhibited the level of MMP-2 by 1%, 15%, 35%, and 67% compared to the untreated control at concentrations of 12.5, 25, 50, and 100 µg/mL (Figure 5A,B), respectively. PSS also exerted an inhibitory effect on the expression of MMP-9. As shown in Figure 5C,D, PSS at a concentration of 100 µg/mL suppressed the expression of MMP-9 by 32%.

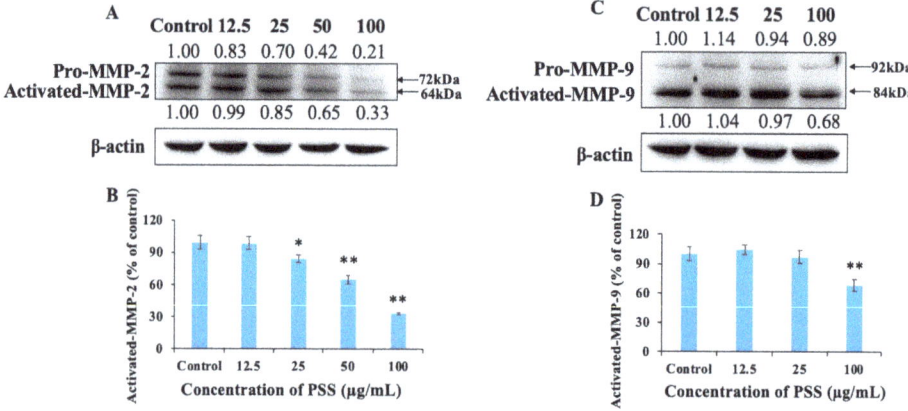

Figure 5. PSS down-regulated the level of activated matrix metalloproteinase 2 (MMP-2) and matrix metalloproteinase 9 (MMP-9) proteins in B16-F10 cells. Cells (2×10^6 cells/dish) were treated with PSS (12.5, 25, 50, 100 µg/mL) for 24 h. Then the cells were harvested, total protein was determined, and SDS-PAGE was performed, as described in the Materials and Methods section. The levels of activated MMP-2 (**A,B**) and MMP-9 (**C,D**) were estimated by Western blotting, also as described in the Materials and Methods section. The numbers underneath the blots represent the band intensities (normalized to the loading controls, means of three independent experiments) measured by ImageJ software (ImageJ 1.8.0, Rawak Software Inc., Stuttgart, Germany). The standard deviations were all within ±15% of the means (data not shown); β-actin was used as an equal loading control. The experiments were repeated three times.

2.6. Propylene Glycol Alginate Sodium Sulfate Decreased the Activity of Matrix Metalloproteinase 2 and Matrix Metalloproteinase 9

We further detected the activity of MMP-2 and MMP-9 in B16-F10 cells after treatment with PSS for 24 h. As shown in Figure 6B,C, PSS inhibited the activity of MMP-2 in a dose-dependent manner. At 25 µg/mL, PSS slightly inhibited MMP-2, while at 50 and 100 µg/mL, it suppressed the activity by 21.8% and 28.7%, respectively. PSS also suppressed the activity of MMP-9 in a similar manner. The inhibition of PSS was 2.7%, 17.2%, and 25.1% at concentrations of 25, 50, and 100 µg/mL, respectively (Figure 6E,F).

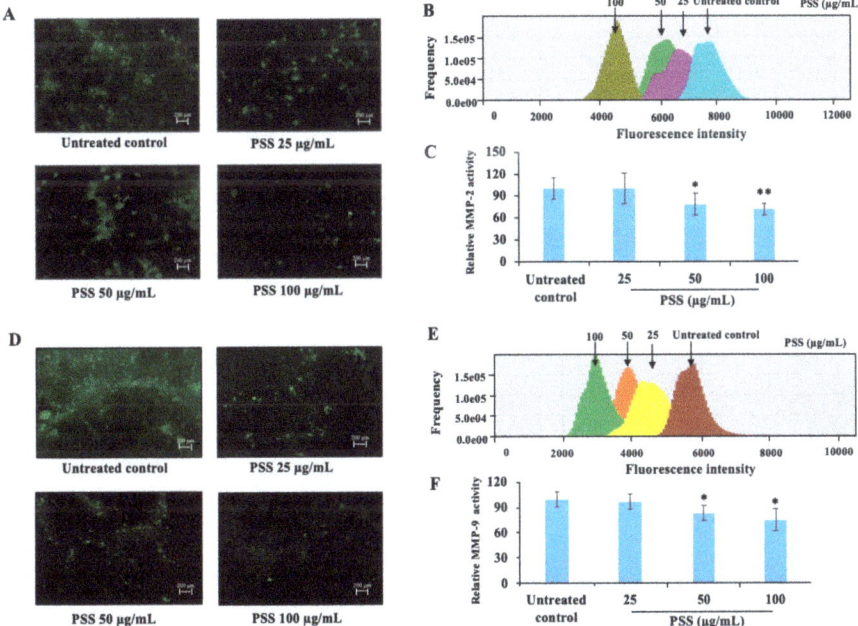

Figure 6. The effect of PSS on the activity of MMP-2 and MMP-9 in B16-F10 cells. The activity of MMP-2 (**A–C**) and MMP-9 (**D–F**) was tested using the GENMED Kit (Genmed Scientifics Inc., Wilmington, DE, USA). Cells (1×10^5 cells/well) were seeded in 12-well culture plates with a glass slide to reach 50% confluence. After being washed with PBS, fresh serum-free culture medium was added to the plate in the presence or absence of serial treatments of PSS (25, 50, 100 µg/mL) for 24 h. The GENMED kit was used to detect the fluorescence intensity. The green dots represent the catalytic sites for MMP-2 or MMP-9, and the fluorescence intensity represents the amount of the degraded gelatin. Fluorescence was visualized in 10 randomly selected fields of view for each cell slide under a fluorescence microscope (Colibri 7, ZEISS, Jena, Germany), and the fluorescence intensity was quantified by ZEN 2.3 lite software (ZEISS, Jena, Germany). The data shown above are from three independent experiments. * $p < 0.05$, ** $p < 0.01$, significant difference between the PSS-treated groups and the untreated control by Student's t-test.

2.7. Propylene Glycol Alginate Sodium Sulfate Down-Regulated the Protein Expression of Vimentin

Carcinoma cells make use of the epithelial–mesenchymal transition (EMT) as they become invasive. Indeed, the transition typically features the loss of cell–cell adherence proteins like cadherin, followed by the loss of apico-basal polarity, and finally, gaining the ability to migrate and invade. To investigate the potential role of PSS in the EMT, two crucial EMT markers in B16-F10 cells were examined by western blot. The expression of Vimentin was decreased by 41% and 47% in the presence of PSS at concentrations of 50 and 100 µg/mL, respectively (Figure 7), while a slight increase was detected in the level of E-cadherin. Additionally, other proteins involved in the regulation of invasion and migration did not show any change in expression after treatment with PSS.

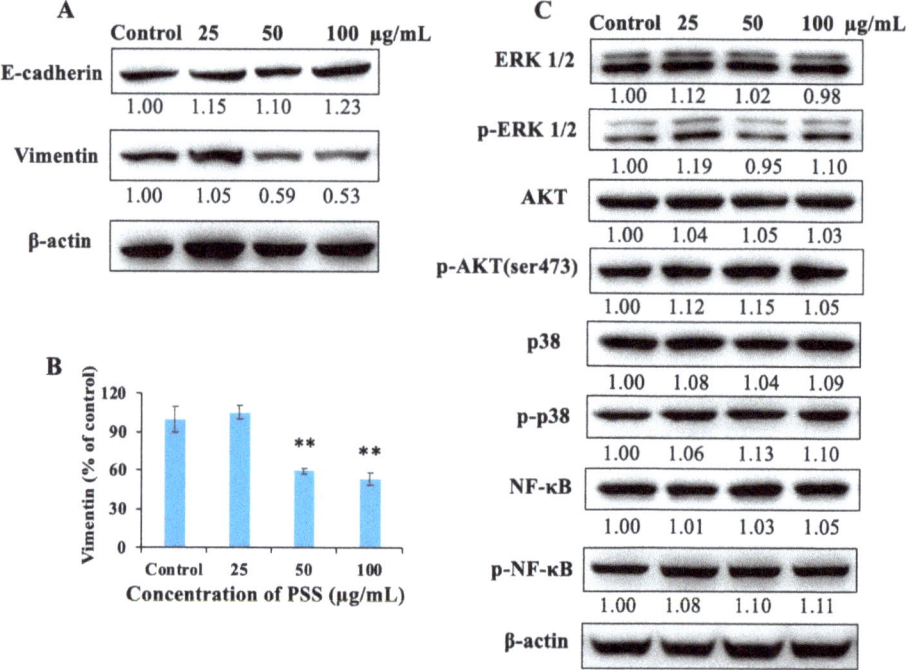

Figure 7. PSS down-regulated the protein expression of Vimentin in B16-F10 cells. Cells (2×10^6 cells/dish) were treated with PSS (25, 50, 100 µg/mL) for 24 h. The cells were harvested, total protein was determined, and SDS-PAGE was performed as described in the Materials and Methods section. The levels of ERK 1/2, p-ERK 1/2, AKT, p-AKT, p38, p-p38, NF-κB, p-NF-κB, Vimentin, and E-cadherin were estimated by Western blotting, as described in the Materials and Methods section. (**A,B**) The protein expression level of Vimentin and E-cadherin in B16-F10 cells. (**C**) The levels of other proteins mentioned above in B16-F10 cells. The numbers underneath the blots represent the band intensities (normalized to the loading controls, means of three independent experiments) measured by ImageJ software (ImageJ 1.8.0, Rawak Software Inc., Stuttgart, Germany). The standard deviations were all within ±15% of the means (data not shown); β-actin was used as an equal loading control. The experiments were repeated three times.

2.8. Propylene Glycol Alginate Sodium Sulfate Inhibited Angiogenesis

We next assessed the capacity of PSS to inhibit angiogenic activity using rat aortic rings and chick chorioallantoic membrane models. As shown in Figure 8A,B, PSS inhibited the outgrowth of new microvessels in a dose-dependent manner. The molecular weight of sulfated polysaccharides including PSS played crucial roles to determine their bioactivities. To illuminate the interaction between molecular weight and anti-angiogenesis potency of PSS, we further detected the effects of PSS fractions with various molecular weights (Mw) (H1: Mw 21.91 kDa; H3: Mw 13.68 kDa; H5: Mw 6.56 kDa; H7: Mw 3.10 kDa; H8: Mw 2.26 kDa) [17] on new blood vessel formation, using the same model. The data showed that the inhibitory effect of the fractions closely correlated with the molecular weight. The H1 fraction (Mw = 21.91 kDa) exhibited the most potent effect among all five fractions, and the inhibitory effect was reduced as the molecular weight decreased (Figure 8C,D). Meanwhile, in the chick chorioallantoic membrane model, PSS suppressed vessel formation at doses of 100 and 200 µg/egg (Figure 8E,F).

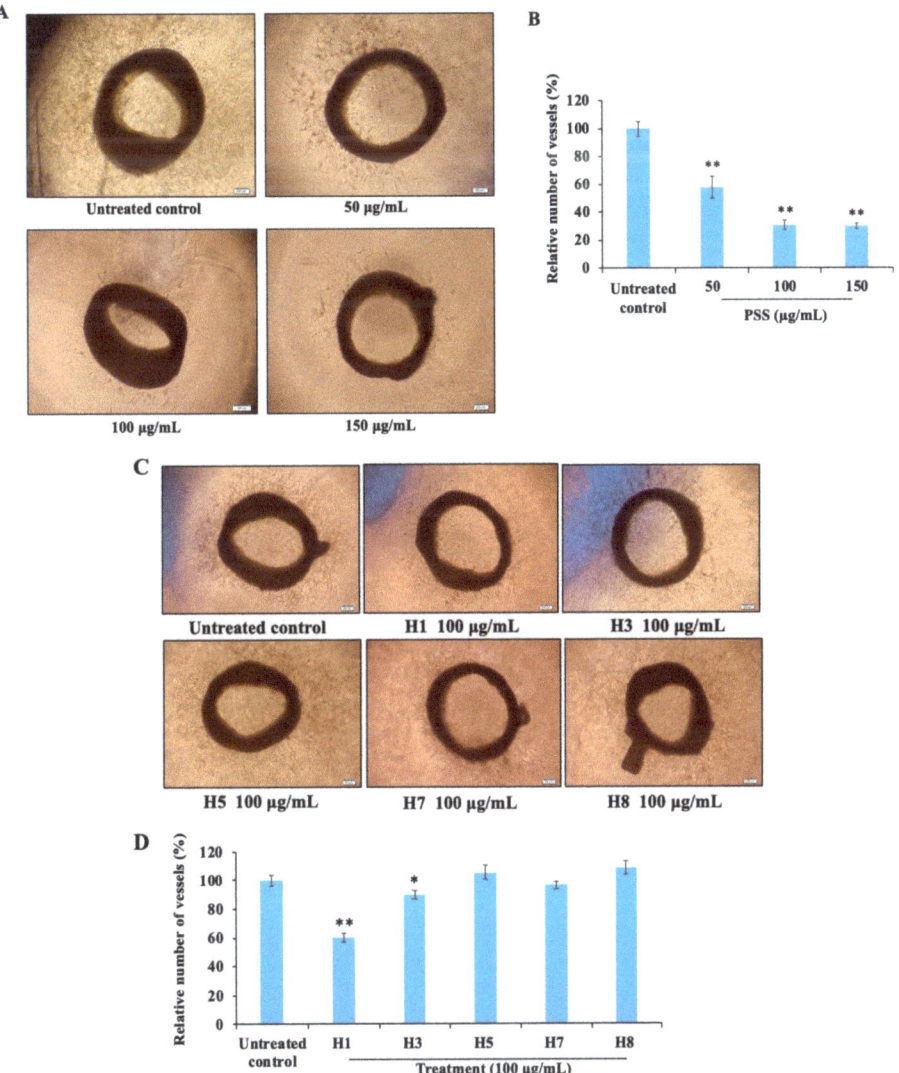

Figure 8. Cont.

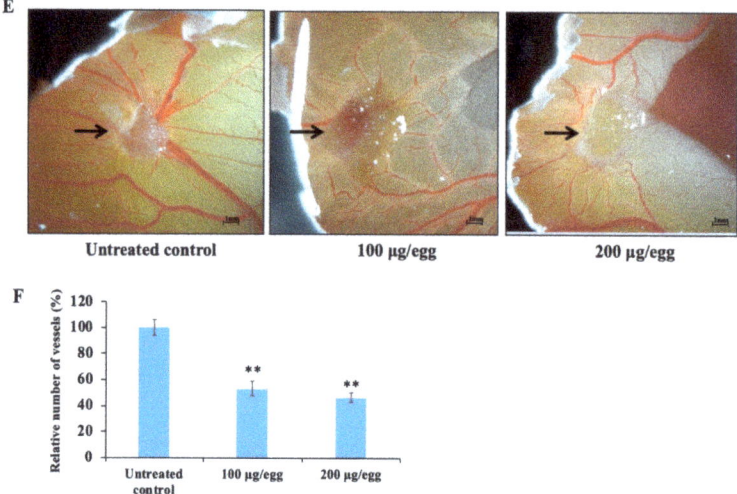

Figure 8. PSS suppresses angiogenesis. The inhibitory effect of PSS on microvessel outgrowth arising from rat aortic rings. Aortic rings were embedded in Matrigel in 96-well plates and then cultured with medium containing various concentrations of PSS (50, 100, 150 μg/mL) for seven days (**A,B**). The effect of fractionated PSS on angiogenesis in the rat aortic ring model. The method used was the same as above (**C,D**). The effect of PSS on angiogenesis in the chick chorioallantoic membrane assay. Gelatin sponges (5 mm × 5 mm) saturated with various concentrations of PSS solution or normal saline were inserted into seven-day-old fertilized eggs (**E,F**). After incubation for another 48 h, the zones of neovascularization under and around the gelatin sponge were photographed under an anatomic microscope (Colibri 7, ZEISS, Jena, Germany) and the black arrows in the photos pointed at the site of gelatin sponge. The total vessel number was quantified by ImageJ software (ImageJ 1.8.0, Rawak Software Inc., Stuttgart, Germany). * $p < 0.05$, ** $p < 0.01$, significant difference between the PSS or PSS fraction-treated groups and the untreated control by the Student's t-test.

2.9. Propylene Glycol Alginate Sodium Sulfate Inhibited Fibroblast Growth Factor 2-Mediated Angiogenesis

To confirm the possible effect of PSS on FGF2-mediated angiogenesis, we cultured rat aortic rings in a serum-free medium, with 200 ng/mL FGF2 in the plate coating with growth factor-reduced Matrigel. As shown in Figure 9, little sprouting was observed in the negative control ring, while substantially more sprouting was observed in the FGF2-treated ring. PSS at 100 μg/mL decreased the level of sprouting to the amount in the negative control, and 200 μg/mL completely suppressed sprouting.

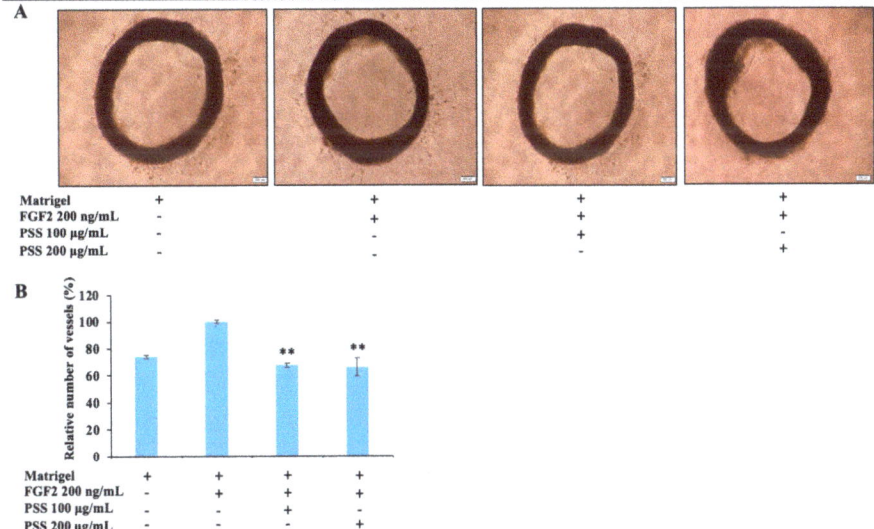

Figure 9. PSS suppresses FGF2-induced microvessel outgrowth in a rat aortic ring model. (**A**) Aortic rings were embedded in growth factor-reduced Matrigel in 96-well plates, and were then cultured with medium containing 200 ng/mL FGF2 and various concentrations of PSS (100, 200 μg/mL) for seven days. Images are representative of three independent experiments with similar results. (**B**) The total vessel number was quantified by ImageJ software (ImageJ 1.8.0, Rawak Software Inc., Stuttgart, Germany). ** $p < 0.01$, significant difference between the PSS-treated groups and the FGF2 control by Student's *t*-test.

3. Discussion

In this study, we observed that PSS has a major impact on invasion and angiogenesis in murine melanoma B16-F10 cells. FGF2 is a proangiogenic factor involved in tumor angiogenesis, invasion and migration. The present findings show that FGF2 bound to PSS with high affinity and inhibited FGF2-mediated angiogenesis in a rat aortic ring model. Moreover, PSS could suppress a FGF2-mediated invasion. The results of a further mechanism study indicate that PSS down-regulated the expression of activated MMP-2 and MMP-9, and also suppressed their activity. In addition, PSS was found to decrease the protein levels of Vimentin, which is known to participate in EMT. Notably, PSS did not elicit any changes in cancer cell viability, even though the concentration was more than 1000 μg/mL.

Previous data indicated that the KD value for heparin binding to FGF2 ranges from 1 to 71 nM [19–22]. These values were affected by a variety of factors, including the method used to determine them, the ionic strength of the buffer, the size and source of the heparin, and the source of the growth factor. In our system, we obtained similar KD values for FGF2 binding to PSS or heparin, indicating that PSS was comparable to heparin in terms of binding to FGF2. We further analyzed the electrostatic potential surface of FGF2. As shown in Supplementary Figure S2, FGF2 displayed a mass area of positive charge in the surface; hence, it could easily bind negative charged compounds. PSS and heparin possess similar sulfate group contents (32.39% and 34%, respectively) and similar KD values to FGF2; therefore, we presume that the sulfate of the two polysaccharides probably accounted for their affinity to FGF2.

FGF2 is known to interact with *N*-sulfoglucosamine (GlcNS) and 2-*O*-sulfated iduronate residues (IdoUA (2S)) in heparin and HS [23,24], but the additional presence of 6-*O*-sulfation is required for biological activity [25,26]. PSS is a heparin-like drug, which is composed of repeating units of mannuronic acid (M) and guluronic acid (G), with 2-*O* and 3-*O* sulfate groups in the sugar rings. Groups that are 2-*O*-sulfated play a crucial role in mediating the binding of heparin with FGF2. Because PSS and heparin exhibited a comparable affinity to FGF2 and, we presume that 2-*O*-sulfated PSS might also be crucial for promoting the interaction of PSS with FGF2. To confirm this presumption, further research should be performed to elucidate the structure–activity relationship.

FGF2 and VEGF165 are the most important growth factors, and can be blocked by heparin to reduce angiogenesis. We also detected the affinity of PSS with VEGF165; however, PSS exhibited weaker affinity to VEGF165 (KD = 1.78×10^{-4} M) than heparin (KD = 8.09×10^{-7} M). Zhao et al. [27] reported that the specific structural features of heparin, such as the content of sulfate, sugar ring stereochemistry, and conformation, determined the affinity of heparin-derived oligosaccharides to VEGF165. Moreover, the positive charge on the surface of VEGF165 was distributed in a dispersed state (Supplementary Figure S2). Based on the above information, we presume that the conformation of PSS might not fit the stereochemical structure of VEGF165.

It was well-documented that the molecular weight of sulfated polysaccharides including PSS played crucial roles in determining their bioactivities. Our previous study showed that the average molecular weight of PSS was about 17 kDa and the distribution range of molecular weight was about 2~20 kDa [17]. Unlike the small molecular compounds, which generally bind to domains with catalytic activity of targeting proteins, sulfated polysaccharides possessed large amount of negative charge and generally interacted with proteins rich in positive potential on the surface of proteins. Theoretically, the longer sugar chains (the higher molecular weight) of the negative charged polysaccharide was endowed with the stronger binding affinity to target proteins and further exerted obvious bioactivities. Here, the higher molecular weight of PSS fractions exerted stronger inhibitory effect on angiogenesis which was consistent with the trend in previous publications [17,28]. Similarly, we speculated that it might be the same trends of PSS fractions in other experiments of the manuscript.

For the first time, we evaluated the effect of PSS on the highly metastatic B16-F10 melanoma cells and the related tumor environment. PSS itself has no inhibitory effect on the growth of B16-F10 cells—however, it suppressed FGF2-mediated angiogenesis and invasion of B16-F10 cells, and also decreased the level of Vimentin, which might help enhance the sensitivity of tumor cells to chemotherapy. Moreover, to fully elucidate the effects of PSS on the tumor microenvironment, further research should be conducted to investigate whether PSS exerts inhibitory effects on other cells involved in the tumor microenvironment, such as endothelial cells, fibroblasts, and immune cells. Meanwhile, further research should be done to combine PSS with chemotherapeutic drugs to check whether a synergistical effect happens.

4. Materials and Methods

4.1. Cell Culture and Reagents

The murine melanoma B16-F10 cell line was all obtained from the Type Culture Collection of the Chinese Academy of Sciences (Shanghai, China). The B16-F10 cells were cultured in RPMI-1640 supplemented with 10% (v/v) heat-inactivated FBS and 1% (v/v) penicillin–streptomycin. HUVECs were obtained from the Procells company (Shanghai, China) and cultured in Ham's F-12K supplemented with 100 μg/mL Heparin, 50 μg/mL ECGs, 10% (v/v) heat-inactivated FBS, and 1% (v/v) penicillin-streptomycin solution. Cells were cultured at 37 °C in a humidified atmosphere containing 5% CO_2. Cells were maintained at subconfluency, and the culture medium was changed every other day. The B16-F10 cells used were between 3 and 30 passages.

PSS was provided by Chia Tai Haier Pharmaceutical Co., Ltd. (Qingdao, China). Heparin (201 U/mg) was obtained from Wanbang Pharmaceuticals Company (Xuzhou, China). All proteins were purchased from Sino Biological (Beijing, China). All antibodies were purchased from Cell Signaling Technology (Cell Signaling Technology Inc., MA, USA). Matrigel was purchased from Corning Company (Tewksbury, MA, USA). All other chemicals and solvents were of analytical grade and purchased from Sinopharm Group Co. Ltd. (Beijing, China)

4.2. The Binding Kinetics of Propylene Glycol Alginate Sodium Sulfate and Fibroblast Growth Factor 2

The kinetics and specificity of the binding between PSS derivatives and FGF2 and VEGF165 proteins were determined by a PlexArray®HT SPR system (Plexera Inc., Seattle, DC, USA). Briefly, PSS (1–5 mM) were immobilized on Graft-to-PCL sensor chips by UV crosslinking for 15 min, according to an established protocol. The mobile phase was FGF2 or VEGF165 solution (dissolved in PBS), and the concentrations used were 125, 250, and 500 nM. The data obtained were analyzed and fitted by PLEXERA SPR DAM to obtain the equilibrium dissociation constant (KD).

4.3. Cell Invasion

Transwell chambers (6.5 mm diameter, 8 μm pore size; Corning Life Sciences) were coated with 100 μL of diluted Matrigel. Then, 0.6 mL of medium containing 10% FBS was added to the lower chambers, and cells suspended in serum-free medium at a density of 1.5×10^5 cells/mL were seeded (0.1 mL) in the upper chambers. Various concentrations of PSS (25, 50, 100 μg/mL) were added to both of the upper and lower chambers. After incubation for 16 h or 8 h (FGF2-mediated invasion of B16-F10), cells were fixed with cold 4% paraformaldehyde and stained with 0.1% crystal violet, and the cells that had not migrated were removed from the upper chambers. The remaining cells were photographed in five random fields per membrane. The dye was dissolved in 80 μL of acetic acid, and the absorbance of the resulting solution was measured at 600 nm using a microplate reader (SpetraMAX i3, Molecular Devices, Sunnyvale, CA, USA).

4.4. Cell Proliferation Assay

B16-F10 cells (0.5×10^4 cells/well) were seeded in 96-well culture plates in 100 μL of culture medium and incubated for 24 h. Subsequently, 100 μL of complete medium without or with various concentrations of PSS (100, 200, 400, 600, 800, 1000 μg/mL) were added. After incubation for 48 h, 10 μL of resazurin solution (1 mg/mL) was then added to each well, and the cells were incubated for another 4 h. The fluorescence of each well was measured at 544 nm and 595 nm by a microplate reader (SpetraMAX i3, Molecular Devices, Sunnyvale, CA, USA).

4.5. Cell Migration

First, 0.6 mL medium containing 10% FBS was added to the lower chamber of Transwell chambers (6.5 mm diameter, 8 μm pore size; Corning Life Sciences), and cells suspended in a serum-free medium at a density of 1.5×10^5 cells/mL were seeded (0.1 mL) in the upper chambers. Then, 400 μg/mL PSS was added to both the upper and lower chambers. After incubation for 16 h, the cells were fixed by cold 4% paraformaldehyde, stained by 0.1% crystal violet, and cells that had not migrated were removed from the upper chambers. The remaining cells were photographed in five random fields per membrane. The dye was dissolved in 80 μL of acetic acid, and the absorbance of the resulting solution was measured at 600 nm using a microplate reader (SpetraMAX i3, Molecular Devices, Sunnyvale, CA, USA).

4.6. The Wound Healing Assay

The effect of PSS on migration was analyzed in vitro using a wound healing assay. B16-F10 cells were seeded in 12-well culture plates to reach 70% confluency. The cell monolayer was scratched vertically down the center of each well with a sterile 200 μL micropipette tip, and rinsed carefully with phosphate buffer solution (PBS) three times to remove cell debris. FBS-free medium with varying concentrations of PSS (100, 400 μg/mL) or 400 μg/mL heparin was added to each well. Three randomly selected views along the wound line in each well were photographed under an inverted microscope at 0 h and 24 h after incubation. The percentage of void area with respect to time 0 was determined using ImageJ software (ImageJ 1.8.0, Rawak Software Inc., Stuttgart, Germany).

4.7. Western Blot Analysis

B16-F10 cells (2×10^6 cells per well) were seeded into a 10 cm dish for 24 h, and then cells were treated with different concentrations of PSS (12.5, 25, 50, 100 μg/mL) for 24 h. The medium was removed, and the cells were washed with PBS three times. Cells were then lysed in 200 μL of lysis buffer on ice. The total protein was determined using the Bicinchoninic Acid (BCA) Kit (Solarbio, Beijing, China). Equal amounts of protein in the cell extracts were fractionated by 10% SDS-PAGE, and then electrotransferred onto polyvinylidene fluoride (PVDF) membranes. After blocking with TBST (20 mM Tris-buffered saline and 0.1% Tween) containing 5% nonfat dry milk for 1 h at room temperature, the membranes were incubated for 2 h with monoclonal antibodies, such as anti-MMP-9, anti-MMP-2, anti-E-cadherin, anti-Vimentin, anti-ERK 1/2, anti-p-ERK 1/2, anti-AKT, anti-p-AKT (Ser473), anti-p38, anti-p-p38, anti-p-p38, anti-NF-κB, anti-p-NF-κB, and anti-β-actin, which were purchased from Cell Signaling Technology. The membranes were then washed three times and incubated with HRP-conjugated secondary antibodies (Abcam, Cambridge, Massachusetts, USA). The proteins were then detected using chemiluminescence agents (Amersham ECL, GE Healthcare, Buckinghamshire, UK).

4.8. In Situ Zymography Localization of Matrix Metalloproteinase 2 and Matrix Metalloproteinase 2 Activity

MMP-2/9 activity was tested on the slides of cells using the GENMED Kit (Genmed Scientifics Inc., Wilmington, DE, USA) according to the manufacturer's instructions (GENMED80062.4/80062.6, GENMED). B16-F10 were seeded in 12-well culture plates with a glass slide until they reached 50% confluence. After washing with PBS, fresh serum-free culture media was added to the plate in the presence or absence of serial PSS treatments, at concentrations ranging from 25–100 μg/mL. After 24 h, the glass slides were carefully removed. Reagent A was heated until melted. Then, 1000 μL of reagent A was transferred into a 1.5 mL microtube and incubated for 10 min at 37 °C in a thermostatic water bath. Reagent B was added to the 1.5 mL microtube and mixed well. The solution was added to the slide, a coverslip was added, and the slide was incubated in the dark at 4 °C for 10 min until the gel solidified. The prepared sections were then incubated at 37 °C for 60 min in the dark. Fluorescence was visualized in 10 randomly selected fields of view for each cell slide at 40× magnification under a fluorescence microscope (Colibri 7, ZEISS, Jena, Germany). The fluorescence intensity of cells with active enzymes of MMP-2 or MMP-9 was quantified by the arithmetic mean intensity of ZEN 2.3 lite software. Each sample was assayed in triplicate, as described previously [29–31].

4.9. Rat Aortic Ring Assay

Aortas were obtained from six-week-old Sprague–Dawley rats. Each aorta was cut into 1-mm slices and washed in sterile PBS three times, and then imbedded into 55 μL of Matrigel in 96-well plates. The aortic rings were then cultured in 100 μL of DMEM medium with 10% FBS and various concentrations of PSS and PSS with different molecular markers. On day 7, the rings were photographed under a microscope (Colibri 7, ZEISS, Jena, Germany). The data obtained were analyzed and quantified using ImageJ software (ImageJ 1.8.0, Rawak Software Inc., Stuttgart, Germany). The animal experiments were approved by the Animal Ethics Committee of Marine Biomedical Research Institute of Qingdao (MBRI-2017-1106), and were strictly followed the guidelines of the institute.

4.10. Chick Chorioallantoic Membrane Assay

Fertilized eggs were incubated in a constant-temperature incubator maintained at 37 °C and 40%–60% humidity for seven days. Gentle suction was applied to the hole located at the broad end of the egg to create a false air sac directly over the chick chorioallantoic membrane (CAM), and a 1–2 cm^2 segment was immediately removed from the eggshell. A round gelatin sponge (5 mm × 5 mm) saturated with PSS solution (100 or 200 μg/egg) or saline was placed into the area between the pre-existing vessels, and the embryos were further incubated for 48 h. The zones of neovascularization under and around the gelatin sponge were photographed under a stereomicroscope (SZX2-ILLT, OLYMPUS). The data obtained were analyzed and quantified using ImageJ software (ImageJ 1.8.0, Rawak Software Inc., Stuttgart, Germany).

4.11. Statistical Analysis

Statistical analysis for in vitro was performed using Excel. A two-tailed Student's unpaired *t*-test was performed to compare the untreated control group with the treated groups. The results were considered significant when $p < 0.05$ (*, $p < 0.05$; **, $p < 0.01$). Independent experiments were conducted with a minimum of two biological replicates per condition to allow statistical comparison. Error bars represent the standard error of the mean, and the *p* values are indicated. All experiments were repeated at least three times.

Supplementary Materials: The following are available online at http://www.mdpi.com/1660-3397/17/5/257/s1, Table S1: Analysis of the affinity between PSS and VEGF165, Figure S1: The effect of PSS on the migration of HUVEC cells, Figure S2: The electrostatic potential surface of FGF2 and VEGF165.

Author Contributions: H.M., P.Q., X.X., M.X., and H.X. performed the experiments. P.Q. designed the experiments. J.Y. and C. L. analyzed data. H.M. and P.Q. wrote the manuscript. J.Y., C.L., and Y.C. revised the manuscript. All the authors approved the final manuscript. All authors discussed the drafts and approved the final manuscript for publication.

Funding: This work was supported by The National Natural Science Fund (Grant No. 31701221), The Marine S&T Fund of Shandong Province for Pilot National Laboratory for Marine Science and Technology (Qingdao) (No.2018SDKJ0404-4), and the Shandong Science and Technology Project (Grant No. 2014GGH215001). Qingdao Leading Talents Program (Grant No. 16-8-3-11-zhc), "Ao Shan Talents" Program Supported by Qingdao National Laboratory for Marine Science and Technology (Grant No. 2017ASTCP-OS11).

Conflicts of Interest: The authors declare that they have no competing financial interests to disclose.

Abbreviations

PSS	propylene glycol alginate sodium sulfate
CAM	chick chorioallantoic membrane
EMT	epithelial–mesenchymal transition
KD	dissociation constant
FGF	fibroblast growth factor
FGF2	fibroblast growth factor 2
FGFRs	fibroblast growth factor receptors
MMP-2	matrix metalloproteinase 2
MMP-9	matrix metalloproteinase 9
SPR	surface plasmon resonance
HS	heparan sulfate
HSPG	heparan sulfate proglycan
M	mannuronic acid
G	guluronic acid
HUVECs	human umbilical vein endothelial cells

References

1. De Aguiar, R.B.; Parise, C.B.; Souza, C.R.; Braggion, C.; Quintilio, W.; Moro, A.M.; Navarro Marques, F.L.; Buchpiguel, C.A.; Chammas, R.; de Moraes, J.Z. Blocking FGF2 with a new specific monoclonal antibody impairs angiogenesis and experimental metastatic melanoma, suggesting a potential role in adjuvant settings. *Cancer Lett.* **2016**, *371*, 151–160. [CrossRef] [PubMed]
2. Rodeck, U.; Melber, K.; Kath, R.; Menssen, H.D.; Varello, M.; Atkinson, B.; Herlyn, M. Constitutive expression of multiple growth factor genes by melanoma cells but not normal melanocytes. *J. Investig. Dermatol.* **1991**, *97*, 20–26. [CrossRef] [PubMed]
3. Rusnati, M.; Presta, M. Fibroblast growth factors/fibroblast growth factor receptors as targets for the development of anti-angiogenesis strategies. *Curr. Pharm. Des.* **2007**, *13*, 2025–2044. [CrossRef]

4. Bikfalvi, A.; Klein, S.; Pintucci, G.; Rifkin, D.B. Biological roles of fibroblast growth factor-2. *Endocr. Rev.* **1997**, *18*, 26–45. [PubMed]
5. Compagni, A.; Wilgenbus, P.; Impagnatiello, M.A.; Cotten, M.; Christofori, G. Fibroblast growth factors are required for efficient tumor angiogenesis. *Cancer Res.* **2000**, *60*, 7163–7169. [PubMed]
6. Itoh, N.; Ornitz, D.M. Evolution of the Fgf and Fgfr gene families. *Trends Genet.* **2004**, *20*, 563–569. [CrossRef] [PubMed]
7. Ibrahimi, O.A.; Zhang, F.; Hrstka, S.C.; Mohammadi, M.; Linhardt, R.J. Kinetic model for FGF, FGFR, and proteoglycan signal transduction complex assembly. *Biochemistry* **2004**, *43*, 4724–4730. [CrossRef]
8. Brown, A.; Robinson, C.J.; Gallagher, J.T.; Blundell, T.L. Cooperative heparin-mediated oligomerization of fibroblast growth factor-1 (FGF1) precedes recruitment of FGFR2 to ternary complexes. *Biophys. J.* **2013**, *104*, 1720–1730. [CrossRef] [PubMed]
9. Jaye, M.; Schlessinger, J.; Dionne, C.A. Fibroblast growth factor receptor tyrosine kinases: Molecular analysis and signal transduction. *Biochim. Biophys. Acta* **1992**, *1135*, 185–199. [CrossRef]
10. Sterner, E.; Masuko, S.; Li, G.; Li, L.; Green, D.E.; Otto, N.J.; Xu, Y.; DeAngelis, P.L.; Liu, J.; Dordick, J.S.; et al. Fibroblast growth factor-based signaling through synthetic heparan sulfate blocks copolymers studied using high cell density three-dimensional cell printing. *J. Biol. Chem.* **2014**, *289*, 9754–9765. [CrossRef] [PubMed]
11. Strutz, F.; Zeisberg, M.; Ziyadeh, F.N.; Yang, C.Q.; Kalluri, R.; Muller, G.A.; Neilson, E.G. Role of basic fibroblast growth factor-2 in epithelial-mesenchymal transformation. *Kidney Int.* **2002**, *61*, 1714–1728. [CrossRef]
12. Liu, J.F.; Crepin, M.; Liu, J.M.; Barritault, D.; Ledoux, D. FGF-2 and TPA induce matrix metalloproteinase-9 secretion in MCF-7 cells through PKC activation of the Ras/ERK pathway. *Biochem. Biophys. Res. Commun.* **2002**, *293*, 1174–1182. [CrossRef]
13. Chung, S.W.; Bae, S.M.; Lee, M.; Al-Hilal, T.A.; Lee, C.K.; Kim, J.K.; Kim, I.S.; Kim, S.Y.; Byun, Y. LHT7, a chemically modified heparin, inhibits multiple stages of angiogenesis by blocking VEGF, FGF2 and PDGF-B signaling pathways. *Biomaterials.* **2015**, *37*, 271–278. [CrossRef] [PubMed]
14. Zeng, Y.; Yang, D.; Qiu, P.; Han, Z.; Zeng, P.; He, Y.; Guo, Z.; Xu, L.; Cui, Y.; Zhou, Z.; et al. Efficacy of Heparinoid PSS in Treating Cardiovascular Diseases and Beyond-A Review of 27 Years Clinical Experiences in China. *Clin. Appl. Thromb. Hemost.* **2016**, *22*, 222–229. [CrossRef]
15. Xue, Y.T.; Ren, L.; Li, S.; Wang, L.L.; He, X.X.; Zhao, X.; Yu, G.L.; Guan, H.S.; Li, C.X. Study on quality control of sulfated polysaccharide drug, propylene glycol alginate sodium sulfate (PSS). *Carbohydr. Polym.* **2016**, *144*, 330–337. [CrossRef] [PubMed]
16. Xin, M.; Ren, L.; Sun, Y.; Li, H.H.; Guan, H.S.; He, X.X.; Li, C.X. Anticoagulant and antithrombotic activities of low-molecular-weight propylene glycol alginate sodium sulfate (PSS). *Eur. J. Med. Chem.* **2016**, *114*, 33–40. [CrossRef] [PubMed]
17. Ma, H.; Qiu, P.; Xin, M.; Xu, X.; Wang, Z.; Xu, H.; Yu, R.; Xu, X.; Zhao, C.; Wang, X.; et al. Structure-activity relationship of propylene glycol alginate sodium sulfate derivatives for blockade of selectins binding to tumor cells. *Carbohydr. Polym.* **2019**, *210*, 225–233. [CrossRef]
18. Wu, J.; Zhang, M.; Zhang, Y.; Zeng, Y.; Zhang, L.; Zhao, X. Anticoagulant and FGF/FGFR signal activating activities of the heparinoid propylene glycol alginate sodium sulfate and its oligosaccharides. *Carbohydr. Polym.* **2016**, *136*, 641–648. [CrossRef]
19. Li, L.Y.; Seddon, A.P. Fluorospectrometric analysis of heparin interaction with fibroblast growth factors. *Growth Factors* **1994**, *11*, 1–7. [CrossRef] [PubMed]
20. Kamei, K.; Wu, X.; Xu, X.; Minami, K.; Huy, N.T.; Takano, R.; Kato, H.; Hara, S. The analysis of heparin-protein interactions using evanescent wave biosensor with regioselectively desulfated heparins as the ligands. *Anal. Biochem.* **2001**, *295*, 203–213. [CrossRef]
21. Lee, M.K.; Lander, A.D. Analysis of affinity and structural selectivity in the binding of proteins to glycosaminoglycans: Development of a sensitive electrophoretic approach. *Proc. Natl. Acad. Sci. USA* **1991**, *88*, 2768–2772. [CrossRef] [PubMed]
22. Cochran, S.; Li, C.; Fairweather, J.K.; Kett, W.C.; Coombe, D.R.; Ferro, V. Probing the interactions of phosphosulfomannans with angiogenic growth factors by surface plasmon resonance. *J. Med. Chem.* **2003**, *46*, 4601–4608. [CrossRef]
23. Faham, S.; Hileman, R.E.; Fromm, J.R.; Linhardt, R.J.; Rees, D.C. Heparin structure and interactions with basic fibroblast growth factor. *Science* **1996**, *271*, 1116–1120. [CrossRef] [PubMed]

24. Turnbull, J.E.; Fernig, D.G.; Ke, Y.; Wilkinson, M.C.; Gallagher, J.T. Identification of the basic fibroblast growth factor binding sequence in fibroblast heparan sulfate. *J. Biol. Chem.* **1992**, *267*, 10337–10341.
25. Guimond, S.; Maccarana, M.; Olwin, B.B.; Lindahl, U.; Rapraeger, A.C. Activating and inhibitory heparin sequences for FGF-2 (basic FGF). Distinct requirements for FGF-1, FGF-2, and FGF-4. *J. Biol. Chem.* **1993**, *268*, 23906–23914.
26. Pye, D.A.; Vives, R.R.; Turnbull, J.E.; Hyde, P.; Gallagher, J.T. Heparan sulfate oligosaccharides require 6-O-sulfation for promotion of basic fibroblast growth factor mitogenic activity. *J. Biol. Chem.* **1998**, *273*, 22936–22942. [CrossRef]
27. Zhao, W.; McCallum, S.A.; Xiao, Z.; Zhang, F.; Linhardt, R.J. Binding affinities of vascular endothelial growth factor (VEGF) for heparin-derived oligosaccharides. *Biosci. Rep.* **2012**, *32*, 71–81. [CrossRef]
28. Stevenson, J.L.; Choi, S.H.; Varki, A. Differential metastasis inhibition by clinically relevant levels of heparins–correlation with selectin inhibition, not antithrombotic activity. *Clin. Cancer Res.* **2005**, *11*, 7003–7011. [CrossRef]
29. Duan, Y.; Zhao, X.; Ren, W.; Wang, X.; Yu, K.F.; Li, D.; Zhang, X.; Zhang, Q. Antitumor activity of dichloroacetate on C6 glioma cell: In vitro and in vivo evaluation. *Onco. Targets Ther.* **2013**, *6*, 189–198.
30. Xin, H.; Liang, W.; Mang, J.; Lin, L.; Guo, N.; Zhang, F.; Xu, Z. Relationship of gelatinases-tight junction proteins and blood-brain barrier permeability in the early stage of cerebral ischemia and reperfusion. *Neural Regen. Res.* **2012**, *7*, 2405–2412. [PubMed]
31. Wang, Z.; Chen, Z.; Yang, J.; Yang, Z.; Yin, J.; Duan, X.; Shen, H.; Li, H.; Wang, Z.; Chen, G. Treatment of secondary brain injury by perturbing postsynaptic density protein-95-NMDA receptor interaction after intracerebral hemorrhage in rats. *J. Cereb. Blood Flow Metab.* **2018**. [CrossRef] [PubMed]

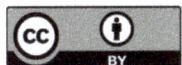

© 2019 by the authors. Licensee MDPI, Basel, Switzerland. This article is an open access article distributed under the terms and conditions of the Creative Commons Attribution (CC BY) license (http://creativecommons.org/licenses/by/4.0/).

MDPI
St. Alban-Anlage 66
4052 Basel
Switzerland
Tel. +41 61 683 77 34
Fax +41 61 302 89 18
www.mdpi.com

Marine Drugs Editorial Office
E-mail: marinedrugs@mdpi.com
www.mdpi.com/journal/marinedrugs